PROFESSIONAL PRACTICE IN SPORT PERFORMANCE ANALYSIS

The use of performance analysis as an evaluative tool in the coaching process is now strongly embedded. This book aims to explore a range of contemporary topics relating to current and future working practices of practitioners in the discipline.

Professional Practice in Sport Performance Analysis delivers practically centred insights into the reality of working in the industry, including the technological, theoretical and personal competencies required. This new book delves into the realities of working as an analyst within the evolving and complex coaching process which practitioners need to navigate in order to successfully deliver their job role. It uncovers the practical realities, underpinning knowledge, challenges and constraints of working as an applied performance analyst whilst providing a practical guide for those practitioners who are currently, or seeking, to work as an applied performance analyst.

Grounded in practice and experience, *Professional Practice in Sport Performance Analysis* helps educate and encapsulate the working realities of the modern-day performance analyst and will be critical reading for students of performance analysis, coaching, skill acquisition and development.

Andrew Butterworth is an experienced applied internationally known performance analyst and academic. His extensive work within netball and badminton spans more than 12 years, including work for the England Netball national team and the Team GB Badminton team. He works closely with elite organisations and clubs to develop the next generation of performance analysts. Andrew is an experienced senior lecturer and programme leader, teaching at Loughborough University, and holds applied consultancy roles with Loughborough Lightning Netball, the Badminton World Federation (BWF) and many others.

Routledge Studies in Sports Performance Analysis

Series Editor: Peter O'Donoghue, Reykjavik University

Routledge Studies in Sports Performance Analysis is designed to support students, lecturers and practitioners in all areas of this important and rapidly developing discipline. Books in the series are written by leading international experts in sports performance analysis and cover topics including match analysis, analysis of individual sports and team sports, technique analysis, data analytics, performance analysis for high performance management, and various methodological areas. Drawing on the very latest research, and introducing key concepts and best practice, the series meets a need for accessible, up-to-date texts at all levels of study and work in performance analysis.

For more information about this series, please visit: https://www.routledge.com/Routledge-Studies-in-Sports-Performance-Analysis/book-series/RSSPA

PROFESSIONAL PRACTICE IN SPORT PERFORMANCE ANALYSIS

Andrew Butterworth

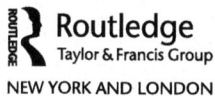

Routledge
Taylor & Francis Group

NEW YORK AND LONDON

Designed cover image: Ben Lumley Photography

First published 2023
by Routledge
605 Third Avenue, New York, NY 10158

and by Routledge
4 Park Square, Milton Park, Abingdon, Oxon, OX14 4RN

Routledge is an imprint of the Taylor & Francis Group, an informa business

ISBN: 978-1-032-12880-1 (hbk)
ISBN: 978-1-032-12879-5 (pbk)
ISBN: 978-1-003-22665-9 (ebk)

DOI: 10.4324/9781003226659

Typeset in Bembo
by codeMantra

For Mia Rose.

CONTENTS

FIGURES

TABLES

FOREWORD

Performance analysis has evolved from notational analysis, as it used to be known. The early work of Mike Hughes and Ian Franks was highly relevant to coaching. Mike Hughes ran the Centre for Performance Analysis at the University of Wales Institute Cardiff (now Cardiff Metropolitan University). The centre provided performance analysis support to teams and individual athletes in many sports through collaboration with both Welsh and British sports governing bodies. Ian Franks developed the Centre for Sports Analysis at the University of British Columbia with the aim of helping athletes improve through the use of feedback on performance within coaching. Both of these centres were also research centres producing pioneering studies into sports performance, but nonetheless the research remained driven by the needs of athletes and coaches in the real world of sport.

From the 1980s to the time of writing (2022), performance analysis has grown considerably both in terms of the volume of work that is being done and in terms of the types of work that are being done. Notational analysis was an appropriate term when shorthand symbols were used to record events using manual systems. The advent of affordable microcomputers allowed computerised notational analysis systems to be developed where shorthand symbols were replaced by function keys or on-screen buttons within graphical user interfaces. It was in 1998 that Keith Lyons introduced the term *performance analysis* at the World Congress of Notational Analysis of Sport IV in Porto. Technology had developed considerably with player-tracking systems being used and video being integrated with match databases in a manner that is now commonplace today within the main commercial video analysis packages. Sports analysis technology has continued to develop at a rapid pace. I can recall writing a book chapter on the use of integrated video and match events that was already out of date by the time the book was published because wireless technology had been added to such systems.

This allowed information to be sent to coaches live during a match as well as multiple analysts using different devices to enter different types of data to the same timeline. There has also been a greater integration with coaching with coaching information systems hosting match videos, statistical information, as well as allowing player and coach discussions about important areas of performance. A further example of the rapid changes in technology was when I saw a former master's student of mine on YouTube using the Hi-Pod camera system at a training venue. I certainly did not teach him how to do that, and it illustrates the need for continuous professional development of analysts to keep abreast of technological and coaching developments.

In some early slides I presented to my students at Ulster University between 2000 and 2003, I made the point that coaching processes should not have to fit in with some performance analysis system but that performance analysis systems needed to support coaching processes. I believed this at the time, but through working as an analyst in netball I have seen how technological advances have allowed coaches to streamline their coaching processes. Maybe I should have seen this coming as there are many types of work, where work processes have changed and improved to exploit new technologies.

The growth of performance analysis within sport has resulted in a performance analysis industry with full-time performance analysts working with clubs and national governing bodies. There remain strong links between universities and industry, but it is a positive development that there is a separate industry to university-based support centres. This is how many industries operate, with the educational establishments preparing students for careers in these industries. Performance analysis is not the only profession where there are strong links between academia and industry. Many major cities have 'university hospitals' where medical practice, research, education and training all take place.

Having established that there is a sports performance analysis industry and that match analysis is a profession, it is clear that there is a need for the book you are currently reading. The early textbooks by Mike Hughes and Ian Franks as well as Chris Carling have certainly covered the development of performance analysis systems to support practical coaching as well as academic research into sports performance. However, when one looks at papers published in the main journal for the area, the *International Journal of Performance Analysis in Sport*, papers on professional practice form a minority of contributions. Such contributions are welcome but, for whatever reason, many researchers prefer to write papers on study sports performance from the outside. This may be due to an inherent bias in research where objective quantitative research may be valued more than more complex qualitative reports. As an editor of the journal, I do find myself disappointed that so many researchers who have access to data from squads they are working with prefer to write up descriptive studies using the data. Many have worked with the clubs and used the data within integrated sports science support teams that serve athletes and coaches. Given that there may still be some scepticism as to whether performance analysis based feedback is effective in helping athletes improve, there is clearly a need for much more in-depth study of performance analysis support within coaching, analyst experiences, as well as coach and player views of performance analysis.

This book is a much welcome contribution to the Routledge Studies of Sports Performance Analysis series. Andrew Butterworth is well positioned to write this book and he has been joined by Luke Gibson, Jon Woodward and myself who have contributed to some of the chapters. I can remember the first time I met Andrew, it was my 50th birthday and Hertfordshire Mavericks were playing Team Bath in the British Netball Superleague. Andrew was an undergraduate at the time, but was using equipment that I'd never used before in working with netball, and he was turning the information around to the coaches in a highly efficient manner. At the time, Hertfordshire University did not have a performance analysis module, but it was an area that Andrew was keen to move and used his dissertation to do so. The dissertation was on practical performance analysis and was published in the *International Journal of Performance Analysis in Sport*. Andrew's work since then has remained driven by practical performance analysis in coaching. As well as working as the Hertfordshire Mavericks analyst as a student, Andrew volunteered to do further work in badminton as well as at the London 2012 Olympics and Paralympics. His PhD was a longitudinal case study of performance analysis support in international netball. Andrew's wealth of experience of working as an analyst has been most beneficial to this book. Andrew has worked with the University of Hertfordshire and Derby University and is now at Loughborough University. I've given an invited lecture to the performance analysis master's programme Andrew teaches on at Loughborough, and all of the students are practising analysts working with clubs or national governing bodies.

This is the first book devoted solely to practising performance analysis and is relevant to all game sports. It is a valuable source of material for practicing analysts in industry as well as aspiring analysts doing work experience modules within universities. This book covers the roles of performance analysts and the skills required. The latest technologies used in the industry are discussed together with the work processes that utilise these technologies. There are different types of analysis done in practice ranging from match to match analysis to longer-term trend analysis and profiling. It also provides insights into how these types of analysis inform coaching. This book provides an honest review of many issues within performance analysis practice, including costs, resource issues, some negative experiences of analysts and the efficacy of performance analysis in helping athletes improve.

Prof Peter O'Donoghue
Reykjavik University, Iceland,
August 2022

PREFACE

Sports performance analysis is one of the most innovative, exciting and techno-logically advanced sports science disciplines. No longer considered the new kid on the block, our discipline is firmly at the forefront of cutting-edge scientific application and decision making in sport. The role has become firmly embedded as a mainstay of interdisciplinary sports science teams globally, within a huge variety of sports, both team and individual. The most popular team sports such as football, basketball and rugby continue to use the discipline heavily as they have done for many years, as do other popular individual sports such as tennis and squash. But now the use of our discipline is also in those sports who previously had little exposure either through choice or lack of resource to provide out-standing support to aid coaches and decision makers in even the most obscure of sports. The growth has also seen analysis transcend the pyramid, working to help enhance youth development, whilst also becoming ever more accessible to non-elite athletes, thanks to affordable and alternative workflows. Even more pleasing is the use of analysis for women's sport which has seen an exceptional and very welcome rise in exposure, professionalism and investment. This is something I am exceptionally proud of and pleased to see, having worked extensively in women's sport including within elite football, badminton and netball.

As a result, this book is written *sport blind*; that is, the content is not directed or focussed in any way to a specific sport, level, gender or other demographic. The text is intended to provide a holistic overview of practicing in the ever-exciting discipline area of sports performance analysis, documenting some of the latest innovations and workflow practices regardless of sport. As the title suggests, this book is intended to be an insight into the practical reality of the knowledge, skills and technologies required to work as a performance analyst. This book provides a hands-on guide, filled with real examples from multiple sports, for those who are currently, or seeking, to work as an applied performance analyst. It uncovers the realities of working as a performance analyst within the evolving and complex coaching process, the range of professional relationships and collaborations that must be developed and navigated, the different technological options available and some of the challenges to the role with some suggested solutions. Meanwhile there is important content about the established value and efficacy of analysis in actually making an impact on the outcome of performance, important content which helps practitioners understand the importance of their job and the direct impacting evidence there is to support its worth.

Critically, this book also explicitly considers you, the practitioner and the emergent needs, development areas and action planning required to forge a successful career in the discipline. This content places a core focus on the practical process of developing skills and knowledge, but also of writing applications, preparing for interviews and knowing how to follow up professionally, whatever the outcome. This book also considers the often overlooked but incredibly important health and safety aspects of performance analysis, centred around a real-life example which served as a call to action for the authors involved to help educate and prevent a similar situation happening to others. Finally, it finishes by considering the financial issues in what can be an expensive discipline, alongside some alternative suggestions for technological investment.

There are many excellent book resources in our area which already provide the underpinning theory, principles and some practical considerations, including those directly in this series of texts. However, there is nothing that discusses the intricacies of the day-to-day realities. This book is that. This is the next step, the practical reality of those underpinnings, on the job, in day-to-day environments, under the intense pressures of sports expectations. Such is the popularity of a career in performance analysis now, this is an important text which helps future and existing practitioners to continually consider their development needs in light of real-world examples and ever-competitive applications. The majority of roles are heavily oversubscribed and it can become frustrating not to get interviewed or appointed, often being left without feedback too. But the good news is that there are also more roles than ever, especially given the investment and use of performance analysis in those areas mentioned just above. That means this book serves as important to help guide you through, provide practical advice and tips and drive your career forwards in our technologically rich, innovative and inspired discipline of sports science.

ACKNOWLEDGEMENTS

Foremost, I'd like to thank Prof Peter O'Donoghue (POD), who has consistently supported me since we first met as rival analysts at a netball game. Soon after, I started my PhD under his expert supervision which was a thoroughly enjoyable experience. POD was critical once again in championing me for this book and helping my initial vision and desire to pursue this become reality, alongside co-authoring a chapter.

To Jon and Luke, who were both fantastic colleagues to work with in my previous job role, thank you for agreeing to take on chapters with me and bringing your substantial expertise to our chapters. Your knowledge has greatly enhanced this text.

Many thanks to Ben Lumley for his outstanding cover photography and other images in this book.

Thanks also go to Hudl, Catapult, Fulcrum, AnalysisPro and Michael Cooper who all kindly provided permission to utilise images, figures and other content resources to bring this book to life. Many thanks also to UK Coaching who kindly provided permission to utilise their resources in Chapter 5.

Finally, to my immediate friends and family who in their various ways helped me immeasurably through the writing of this book, despite a period of immense personal challenge. That period has taught me more about myself than I ever knew possible, and the incredible strength and resilience that brings.

CONTRIBUTORS

Andrew Butterworth Loughborough University, UK.

Peter O'Donoghue Reykjavik University, Iceland.

Jon Woodward University of Derby, UK.

Luke Gibson University of Derby, UK.

1

PERFORMANCE ANALYSIS IN THE COACHING PROCESS

Andrew Butterworth and Jon Woodward

Introduction

Considering the performance analysis directed nature of this book, starting with a focus on coaching might seem strange or questionable to some, wondering if you picked up the correct book. However, the reasoning is simple; to become a better analyst you have to better understand coaching, and vice versa. As a discipline of sports science, performance analysis is part of a complex web of inter-relating disciplines, involving multiple technologies, techniques and intricacies. Myriads of people complicate this already messy process further, each bringing their own philosophies, ideas and experiences to try and deliver support to the ultimate end users. Psychological, sociological and physiological factors are rife within this environment and develop a vast ecosystem in which coaches attempt to undertake their work filled with complex and contextual considerations (Butterworth et al., 2013). If we as performance analysis practitioners are to undertake our own roles successfully and deliver outstanding support to coaches and athletes in this space too, it would be remiss of us to not think that we need to take time to invest in learning some of the intricacies of this environment, and how to operate within them in a holistic manner to better support our end users. Owing to this, this book starts by considering critical questions about what coaching actually is, what the coaching process is and how analysts can seek to support this by providing objectivity, clarity and information within those confines. New research and evolving thoughts about the nature of coaching are constant, with over 1,000 publications to date in the area having been critically considered. So that direct focus and relevance is found in this text, content here is focussed in and around the nature of coaching and the coaching process in direct relation to the role and place of performance analysis, which holds extreme importance and a growing stature. Wright et al.'s (2016) research confirms the

DOI: 10.4324/9781003226659-1

widespread use of performance analysis within the coaching process, yet simultaneously confirms that little consideration is given to the context which surrounds it and the impacts back to players, and so this chapter aims to address this, in an applied and practically centred chapter which seeks to enhance knowledge about the process and provide practical implementation tips for use.

Defining Coaching and the Coaching Process

Providing a simple definition of coaching is not easy, if we were to attempt to in a single word we might elect for *messy*, in another we might go for *ambiguous*. Despite a huge number of publications into the discipline, it is acknowledged that there is not a consensual definition of the discipline that sits at the heart of sport. As Butterworth et al. (2013) explained, early definitions of coaching were criticised as being too simplistic and not representing the true nature, for example Miles' (2003) work which suggested that coaching was simply the development and improvement of people. In an attempt to address the simplification, research was undertaken to meta-analyse definitions towards a consensus and key definitions phrases, elaborating towards multidimensionality and uncertainty amongst others (Cushion & Lyle, 2010). This lack of consensus, characterised by complications in words of definition is perhaps not surprising though since the nature of coaching is so multifaceted, driven by social interactions and micro-political issues. Each of these elements (amongst others) brings a unique and dynamic being to the conceptualised nature of coaching, and as further moving parts are added in, it is not hard to see why a consensual definition is still lacking. From their study in 2011, Abraham and Collins discovered that despite articles being published in an attempt to dissect and understand it better, the very definition and nature of coaching is still under discussion and interpreted differently by different coaches. Since this observation, more research has been published with still no agreed consensus around the definition and nature of coaching, and its many associated facets, that the coaching industry can agree on and work to. But accepting these complexities and acknowledging the multifaceted nature of coaching, given the dynamic nature of the sporting ecosystem perhaps the time has come to step away from obsessing about singular definitions and instead focus attentions towards how practitioners in all disciplines can seek to work within these confines, delivering clarity of place for coaches, and the coaching process, of discipline specific best practice.

This coaching process is the conceptual 'place' where coaching takes place. Here, the coach takes in and absorbs information from multiple sources and disciplines before making decisions on which information to transmit, which steps to take and which methods to utilise in presenting back to the ultimate end users, the athletes. Lyle (2002) considers that this coaching process should be co-ordinated and planned, and should be integrated into a programme for competition, whilst Borrie and Knowles (2003) identified it is a set of stages that a coach navigates in order to help educate and develop their performers. These are just two definitions from literature with the majority of descriptions of the coaching process from researchers often drawn from authors own previous experiences of practical coaching in different environments. This again creates confusion towards a singular definition given that so many personal preferences and biases will influence any new definition. Cushion (2007) recognised that existing definitions of the coaching process had not considered the increasing complexity of the coaching process in practice and the related impact of the sub-elements as contributing factors. And so as with coaching itself, whilst we are no nearer to a consensual definition, what we do agree upon is that the coaching process is the cycle of events in which broad, messy and non-linear decisions are made, driven by social interactions and other contextual factors (Franks et al., 1983; Lyle, 1999; Groom et al., 2011; Mackenzie & Cushion, 2013).

Coaching Process Models

Many models of this cyclic representation of the coaching process have been put forward by researchers in an attempt to provide a graphical overview of it, linked to the stages of delivery in a match-to-match cycle. There are two widely accepted types of model put forward in this regard, those *for* the coaching process and those *of* the coaching process. Models *for* the coaching process are idealistic representations of what coaching practice looks like, arising from assumptions and pre-set beliefs which do not draw upon empirical practice and expert interpretations. This is problematic as the models make a number of assumptions about practice and appear to position coaching as a series of mechanical steps through which practice happens, rather than placing coaching in its messy reality (Cushion et al., 2006). Meanwhile, models *of* the coaching process have been developed in situ with empirical research and an analysis of expert coaches delivering and undertaking their roles. These models provide a more realistic representation of the coaching process, since they have been drawn from actual coaching practice in authentic sport scenarios. These models, whilst not perfect and immune from criticism, attempt to reflect the more complex reality of coaching in practice, seeking to examine practitioner's knowledge, strategies and relationship building tendencies.

It is important that we understand both types of these models, as they are useful in helping us understand the role of coaching, and lead us towards a fuller understanding of the coaching decisions that are made and the complexities involved. Hence, here we'll start to examine some of the models, making note if they are *for* or *of* the coaching process, and considering some criticisms of each in line with the practical reality of the world coaches (and analysts) operate in. Early iterations of coaching process models provide very simple schematics and representations of coaching, reducing its complexity into what appears to be presented as a series of simple steps. They make little to no mention of any support disciplines either, including performance analysis, which is far from the reality of how coaches operate today. The most basic of these concepts is often the one most widely utilised especially in initial learning, penned simply as 'Plan, Do, Review', and has formed the basis of some sports coaching discussion for decades (Figure 1.1). Each of these stages documents the elements of the process that occurs, yet despite laying a good foundation for the actions that can be taken in the coaching process, it is extremely vague and lacks any context or description as to what may occur within each section. Miles (2003) believes that these three stages underpin the coaching process due to the coach's roles in influencing and developing their participants whilst also creating an appropriate environment for this to occur.

In the applied practice of coaching, however, there needs to be the consideration of several more complex iterations developed from this simple three step process, embracing wider contextual and behavioural concepts. With this in mind, Franks et al. (1983, cited in Dancs & Kovacs, 2019) developed and designed a model for coaching (Figure 1.2), which described what a coaching process could look like in applied practice considering performance analysis, developing on from the simple three stage concept but following a similar pattern to the Plan, Do, Review model (Figure 1.1). It develops the idea of the continuous cycle of the process, with the idea of a fluid, reoccurring path with additional considerations (e.g. accounting for past results), and makes a first mention of a form of performance analysis. This also has no defined start and end elements assigned though in a logical process in practice, there are more obvious 'start' points which are relevant to support the planning and reflective processes. Miles (2003) confirms this, that the coaching process in this set can begin at any point within a cycle, with the understanding that different stages may overlap or merge into each other, causing a more collaborative or wider approach.

Whilst it would appear that the model suggests that the coaching process is a structured and organised system to follow, in reality it is not a rigid and formulaic process. Characterising coaching in a two-dimensional model such as this appears to promote the view of coaching as a sequential composite of logical episodes, consequently mis-representing the complexity of actions, relationships and interactions, failing to unearth the functional intricacy that lies beneath (Jones & Wallace, 2005; Cushion, 2007). The same might also be said about models *for* the coaching process developed by Fairs (1987) and Sherman et al. (1997), who both presented coaching as a transactional chain of events with little

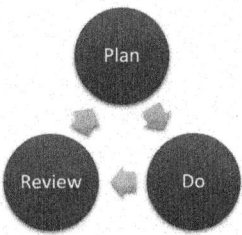

FIGURE 1.1 The 'Plan, Do, Review' coaching process model.

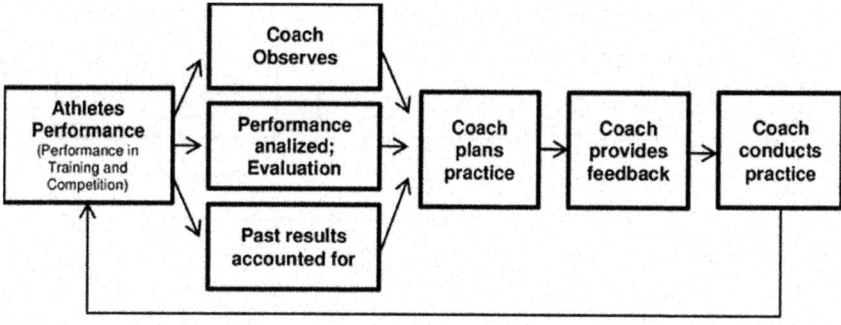

FIGURE 1.2 Franks et al.'s (1983, cited in Dancs & Kovacs, 2019) model *for* the coaching process.

to no consideration paid to any impacting variables. Not surprisingly, despite its logical state and steps which do give a basic guide to steps involved in coaching, the Fairs (1987) model has been criticised for its simplicity and failing to recognise the complexities of performance, the dynamic nature of relationships and lacks practical reality, all void of context (Cushion et al., 2006). The Sherman et al. (1997) model attracts similar criticism from Cushion et al. (2006), who state that the model attempts to place coaching as an instruction model in a series of episodes, again reducing its complexity in practice.

In reality, the coaching process is filled with numerous micropolitical issues and external influences that may have to be managed at multiple stages (Butterworth et al., 2013). As Cushion (2007) has already recognised, the development of previous models such as these do not take into consideration other wider influencing and contributing factors, which will, in practice, limit the effectiveness of the coaching process in applied settings. This mirrors the coaching approach as a whole and underpins that whilst models are representative of the process, it is far from a linear structured process and is inherently messy and disordered at times. Another criticism of these and other such models is that they appear to be structured to prepare for short-term issues or goals and lack any direction or mention of long-term goals when constructed. Existing literature and examples of coaching processes do not contain any suggestions towards long-term planning due to the simplicity of the descriptions (Cushion, 2007; Butterworth et al., 2013). This may be problematic as placing coaching in such a single iteration, rather than paying wider attention to the long-term impacts and multiple cycles of preparation and delivery, promotes the view of siloed work rather than collaborative and holistic approaches. It is also argued that models such as those examined so far fail to distinguish between performance and participation levels of coaching, whilst also failing to consider the relationships that develop between coaches, staff and athletes (Cushion et al., 2006).

Models *of* the coaching process are developed based upon an analysis of coaches actual practice before being diagrammed, with the models typically more widely accepted as useful for practice since they are based on actual practice. MacLean

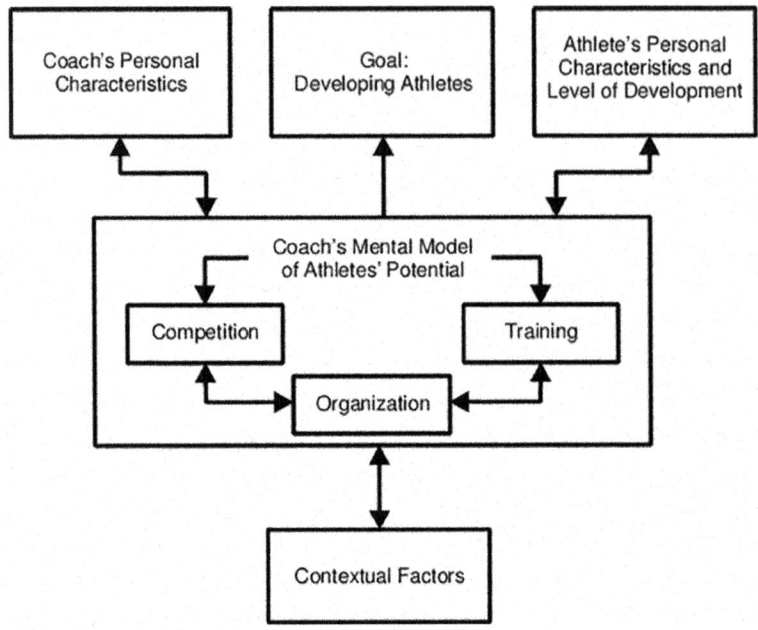

FIGURE 1.3 Cote et al.'s (1995) model *of* the coaching process.

and Chelladurai (1995) and D'Arripe-Longueville et al. (1998) both present models *of* the coaching process having collected empirical data and modelled in a schematic. Cote et al. (1995) meanwhile present a model *of* coaching which is based upon observation and empirical research initially using expert gymnastics coaches as the sample population. The outcomes resulted in a model (Figure 1.3) considering the importance of coach – athlete interaction, as well as additional personnel and contextual factors. The model develops the four elements of training, organisation, competition and potential in turn, which it could be argued accounts for earlier criticisms of performance vs. participation, with a nod towards talent identification and development. The model too also proposes taking into account the coaches own style and interpretation, the athlete themselves and the varying contextual factors that impact upon performance with the overall goal of considering the development and nurturing of the athlete(s). Though this model too is not void of criticism, with Cushion et al. (2006) concluding the inability of the authors to transfer this complexity observed in practice, into the findings of the research, which still places coaching practice as a simplistic schematic, lacking dynamism.

In all of these models what is consistently recognised is the ultimate aim to provide onward information to performers with a view to a superior performance occurring. Research from Gutiérrez-Aguilar et al. (2016) suggests that this might be the case in practice, having undertaken empirical research which suggests that positive performance actions increase in the moments directly after reinstruction and interactions from coaches, with visible structural changes evident. This helps us rationalise the importance of coaching practice and of coaches' roles, with clear evidence to show that coaching does work and does make an impact on the performance of athletes if their messaging is accurate and reliable. It is here though that we hit a snag and our first problematic issue is apparent. Sport is exceptionally dynamic; there are a huge number of contextual impacting factors, including the opposition, venue, time of day and score line to name but a few, with each of these having potential impact on the outcome of a performance and the analysis of a performance. Given this, it is impossible for coaches to success-fully recognise, interpret and consider these in real time when delivering their feedback, it is also impossible for them to recall every single moment within a game. The human brain has limitations and naturally, coaches forget things, no matter the number of notes taken. The amount of information that coaches successfully recall from training and matches varies hugely, with some favoura-ble estimates suggesting 59% of critical events are recalled (Wright et al., 2012). Lacking full recall ability means that there is a lack of accuracy in decision mak-ing, whereby a coach's perception of performance and their subsequent decision making, becomes distorted by those events that they can, or cannot remember (Hughes & Bartlett, 2008). This means that there is a huge deficit or inaccuracy in knowledge and means that void of any support to help this, coaches make de-cisions based off just a fraction of the overall picture.

Performance Analysis' Role

To provide more accurate feedback and to deliver critical insights with a fuller picture, that information deficit must be plugged. Thankfully, performance anal-ysis has been recognised as a tool that can help with that, with research consist-ently providing empirical backing for the vital and pivotal role that the discipline should play in the coaching process. For example, the works of Thelwell (2005) and Groom et al. (2011) recognise performance analysis as integral to success, and essential for behaviour modification. The importance of observation, analy-sis and feedback lies at the heart of the coaching process, with feedback deemed critical to success, and so given that performance analysis provides unbiased and objective feedback, it is seen as an advocate to coaching practice (Carling et al., 2005; Mayes et al., 2009; Butterworth et al., 2013).

So entwined are the roles of feedback and communication in both coach-ing and performance analysis, a collaborative learning approach is critical to the development of enhanced performance outcomes moving forwards. With the ongoing advent of wider academic research and influence within the coaching process, it should not be surprising that the influence of performance analysis has emerged to play a more significant role of informing the coach and helping to manage the coaching process (Francis & Jones, 2014). Wright et al. (2013) state the relevant observation and the ability to assess performance are considered primary roles of a coach and it should be considered to be crucially important within any level, environment and context of sport and performance for the coach to have the ability to evaluate their own athletes' performances and provide feedback appropriate corrective feedback (Nelson & Groom, 2012; Fernandez-Echeverria et al., 2019). This is key area of influence that the more sustained and relevant use of performance analysis can be developed further as a support mechanism within the coaching process, as it allows for an objective interpretation of the complex reality of performance and the environment in which performance improvement occurs (Butterworth et al., 2013; Fernandez-Echeverria et al., 2019). Furthermore, O'Donoghue and Mayes (2013) suggest that performance analysis can act as a superglue, binding together different information sources, which promotes an exciting opportunity for coaches to make use of our critically informed, objective and collaborative discipline for their successes. Empirical studies embedded within multiple different sports agree too, with other chapters of this book explicitly dedicated to deeply understanding the role and value of analysis in applied settings, highlighting some excellent research which portrays the value performance analysis brings to practice.

With the obvious recognition of varying descriptions and definitions of performance analysis, each maintains that it provides objectivity, informed insights and aids recall. That is critical for the role of performance analysis in coaching, helping to provide coaches with more information that is better in accuracy, usability and specificity, a core remit of the discipline in practice. It is crucial that coaches that choose to integrate performance analysis into their coaching process have access to accurate and reliable sources to avoid and eradicate the possibility of subjectivity in the feedback process (Knudson & Morrison, 2002). Not only this, but access to the appropriate technology to use performance analysis has been suggested to improve and facilitate the learning and understanding surrounding certain aspects of performance in coaching (Bampouras et al., 2012; Fernandez-Echeverria et al., 2019). This, and other past literature in performance analysis, has run at times in parallel with coaching, focussing on the practical implementation of our discipline to enhancing performance outcomes, though primarily focussing on *what* it provided, rather than *how* to provide it (Butterworth et al., 2013). This chapter, and indeed this book as a whole, responds to that and considers *how* to provide the best analysis practice for use within the coaching process. Knowledge gained so far about the intricacies of coaching is the first step in that, as we now start to consider the practical place and role of performance analysis at the varying stages of the coaching process through a discussion of some of the models which explicitly consider the two disciplines in tandem.

Modelling Performance Analysis in Coaching

Different models in a variety of sports have been considered from an *of* perspective to deliver schematic representations and overviews of the close relationship and working practices of performance analysis and coaching together. Duckett

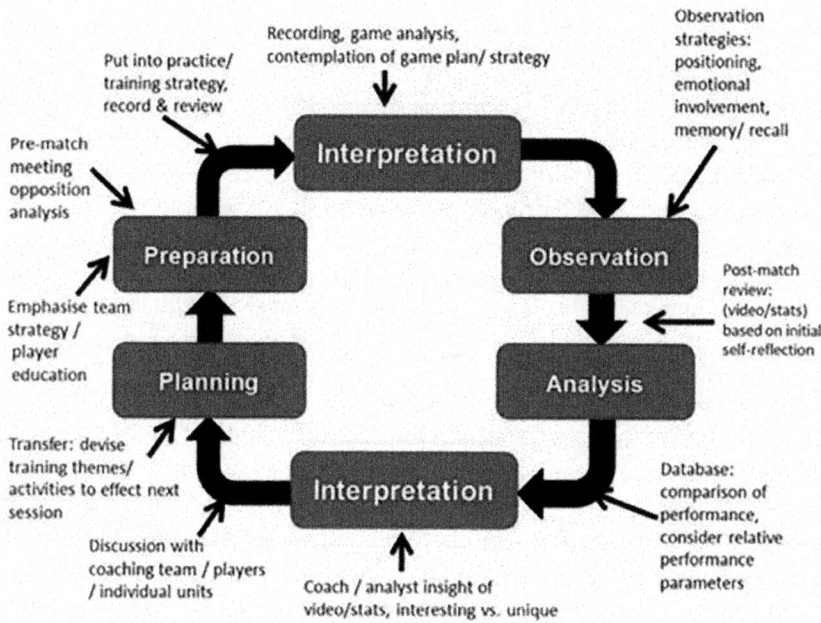

FIGURE 1.4 Duckett's (2012) model of the coaching process. Adapted from Carling et al. 2005; cited in Wright et al., 2014.

(2012) provided an adapted version of Carling et al.'s (2005, cited in Wright et al., 2014) model to deliver a detailed look into the role of performance analysis in the coaching process (Figure 1.4). The adaptation was made to consider how a single cycle looks, when including and considering the roles of pre- and post-match analysis amongst others. In contrast to Cushion's (2007) views regarding earlier models surrounding the coaching process being too simplistic, the Duckett adaptation expands on the basic three step process and uncovers preparation, observation and evaluation / diagnosis as key use areas of analysis directly within coaching, though these do bear remarkable similarities to the 'Plan, Do, Review' model earlier discussed. What is different is the suggested performance analysis elements at each stage of the coaching process, offering useful insight of where the most impactful intervention is perceived to be, with it also worth noting that some elements sit fluidly in-between stages. To this end, although not modelled in a schematic, Sarmento et al.'s (2015) research in futsal uncovers the specific areas in which performance analysis helps within the coaching process and highlights that match analysis, characterised most commonly by video analysis, is the most popular use area. This cements the role of analysis within coaching, helping coaches to make more informed in-game decisions during the 'live' part of delivery within matches. It is also a lean towards the use of video and further backup to the findings established previously by Wright et al. (2012) through their qualitative data collection mechanisms in empirical environments.

The model places our discipline as a key element within all stages, as well as in between and across the stages. Whilst this presents a useful diagrammatic representation of some of the stages performance analysts will be involved with, it simplifies the role of analysis significantly into a linear process and does not consider any flux or unexpected situations to occur. In reality, analysts are asked by coaches to change or adapt work at very short notice, scrapping work they may have just spent a week or more on in favour of a new project, or they are presented with a change in the opposition line up due to injury at last minute and have to provide unexpected new knowledge at exceptionally short notice. None of this unpredictability is considered here and much like the earlier models of coaching, the suggestion of a linear path could not be farther from the truth for analysis practitioners. Furthermore, it provides no detail regarding the *who* or *how* aspects, including no mention of the plethora of technologies (and money) required in order to navigate this suggested analysis workflow or the human re-source and significant training required to operate a successful system.

Further empirical models of performance analysis and coaching come in elite netball research. Horne (2013; Figure 1.5) centred a version around an expanded Plan, Do, Review concept, but further identified key performance analysis components to support at each. The additional key element is the continuous

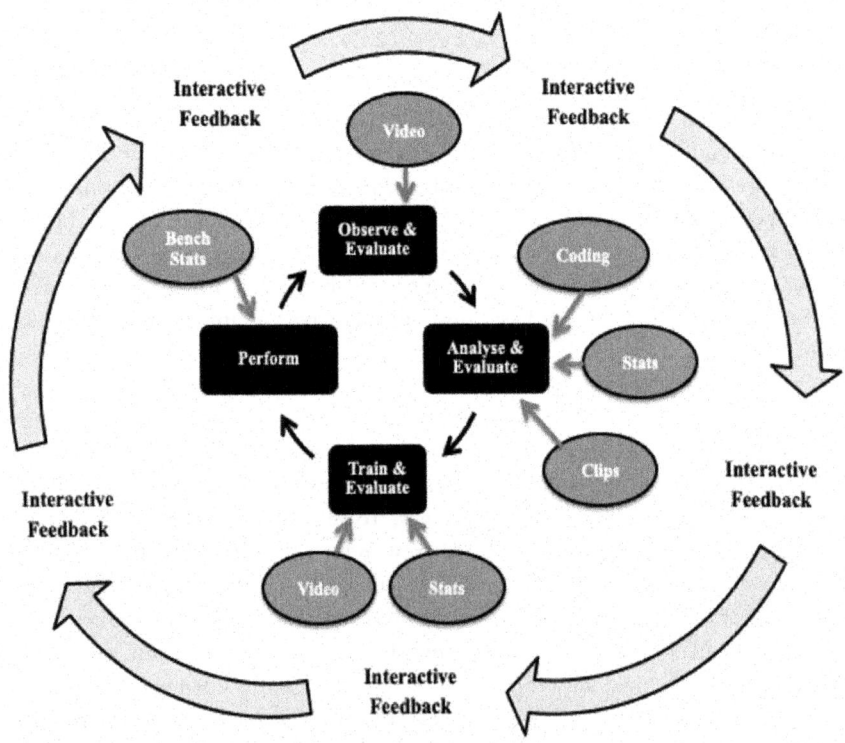

FIGURE 1.5   Horne's (2013) model *of* performance analysis in coaching.

'Interactive Feedback' that encircles the model, with the emphasis on target setting and communication within the multidisciplinary team being crucial throughout the process, a welcome nod towards cross-discipline working. Though useful to model, the performance analysis suggestions lack any form of detail and are too broad and generic to be useful for practice, e.g. 'clips' is very vague and makes no suggestion of which clips, what indicators or how they will be presented. Given the flux of new technologies into the discipline and exceptionally advanced workflows, this is remiss and means the model lacks applicability to wider environments.

Mayes et al. (2009, cited in O'Donoghue & Mayes, 2013; Figure 1.6) consider a cyclic process with the process being player-centred, a positive step which is important since the ultimate recipients of coaching and analysis are the players themselves, also mirroring the very purpose of coaching as a whole. The model identifies further stages to work through than other simpler models and more details about the role of analysis at each, which does help provide a more coherent view of the complexities and multiple roles an analyst will have to undertake. Information flow is also considered which is largely two way for the best part,

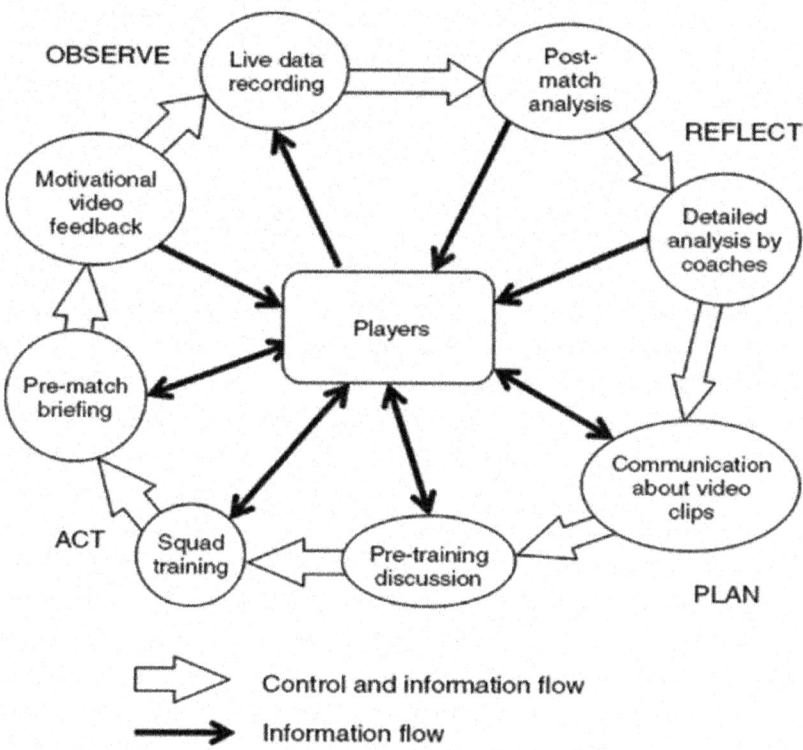

FIGURE 1.6 Mayes et al.'s (2009, cited in O'Donoghue & Mayes, 2013) model *of* performance analysis in coaching.

though some elements lack critical conversation with players such as post-match analysis, which does not reflect the majority of coaching environments, especially given the shift towards player-led responsibility and ownership of performance.

Overall, all models are attempting to represent the coaching process as well as some considering the relational aspects with the majority of existing models of coaching and performance analysis depicted as a cyclic process, with no recognised start or end point. Coaching is a web of complex, context-dependent activities that together form the holistic coaching process and it can be suggested that whilst the models do follow a distinctive, logical order, these individual loops are part of a continuous chain of loops where the processes are repeated, often multiple times at once. It would also be naïve to consider it is a clear linear process, and whilst there appears to forward motion through the stages, with the inherent concept of coaching being non-linear, movement along the cycle might involve moving backwards, or even missing out stages in the light of new information, interpretation or unexpected developments. This is the true dynamism of coaching and the excitement and innovation of performance analysis.

Does This Matter, Anyway?

In spite of theories, models and schematics, in reality coaching and performance analysis are two very practical disciplines. Academic theory and models such as these often feel very far away from the frenetic and fast-paced world of sport and the quick decisions that have to be made. In reality, many coaches do not base their decisions or practice on theory, instead basing their practice on feelings, intuition, 'gut' and previous experiences which trigger coaching decisions (Cross, 1995; Saury & Durand, 1998; Gilbert & Trudel, 2001; Cushion et al., 2003; Jones et al., 2004; Butterworth et al., 2013). Meanwhile Cushion (2007) also states that it would be naïve to believe that all coaches stick to their own process or have considered their actions as a coach to be 'following a process', emphasising that the coaching process will be interpreted differently by each individual coach, meaning the role of analysis may change too. The same largely applies for performance analysis too, with research establishing that performance analysis is poorly defined and lacking any form of conceptual framework to help guide practitioners, leaving a feeling of uncertainty and a lack of structure for practice (Wright et al., 2014). Though, this is challenged with contemporary research from Martin et al. (2021) who identified the importance of building relationships within the professional environment as one of five key components and thus attempted to construct a valid framework for performance analysts to follow.

And so, given the lack of definitions, structure or frameworks, you'd be forgiven for wondering if any of what you have just read actually matters. Well, it does. Because the two disciplines are so tightly entwined and because the role of analysis is so well embedded within coaching practice and the process of coaching, that knowledge gained here will be critical for the ongoing development of analysis skills and practice with the ultimate goal of increasing end performance.

It matters too because knowing the messy and unpredictable nature of coaching is important to understand for working analysts, without longing for exact structure and certainty in process which will likely never come. Knowing how coaching operates and some of the stages involved, alongside the decisions coaches themselves have to make will shape analysis practice and decisions that are made. It is also critical so that analysis practitioners can help educate and inform coaches as to the value and benefits that performance analysis brings. Despite evidence to promote its worth and value, not all coaches will buy into the discipline. Some may have pre conceived ill-defined perceptions which are drawn from their own previous experiences of playing or coaching through different environments, whilst some generations may see the discipline as a form of threat to their own job role (Butterworth et al., 2012). It is this experience which presents a challenge to us as analysts as we must be mindful of this and ensure that the coaches' we work with have had relevant training, experience and an understanding of the usefulness that performance analysis technology might bring (O'Donoghue & Mayes, 2013; Kraak et al., 2018; Painczyk et al., 2018). An increased appreciation and understanding of coaching and coaching structures, alongside an appreciation that performance analysis is not a discipline working in silo, gained through this chapter and other excellent resources should aid that, and move coaches towards a holistic understanding of the usefulness and impact of our discipline in practice.

Practical Considerations

In this chapter, we have unpicked many important aspects of coaching practice, linking directly to the role that performance analysis plays. For performance analysts, there are a host of practical realities that much of this theory and modelling will present itself as in practice. It is important that we unpick this content further and consider some of the potential scenarios that may become apparent as part of the coaching process so that practitioners can consider their potential responses. Linking back to the models we have already reviewed here, there are various steps considered which may occur in every day practice. The content does not seek to provide bespoke solutions or exact suggested responses to practitioners, rather give a trigger of thought for the individual to have critical reflection opportunities about their personal and professional reactions to develop alongside some generalisable suggestions. This seems an appropriate approach, given that every scenario in every different sport and environment has a multitude of evolving and dynamic factors. It would therefore be illogical and inappropriate to suggest a single one-size-fits-all approach to each given the dynamism of evolving situations.

Through the use of performance analysis, there is the potential for a large amount of information that can be utilised by the coach to support the coaching process, but one of the drawbacks could be around how much time and willingness the coach has to fully utilise the information and its potential impact. Time is critical in many aspects of sport, not least when considering the turnaround time between training sessions or games and the desire from end-users to have accessible information. If information is delayed, then this may provide issue for coaches' delivery of sessions or movement to the next stage of their coaching process. Analysts must then consider firstly if they know what these time pressures are and engage in conversations with coaches and other practitioners who should also be reasonable and understanding about sensible agreed turnaround times, before then considering the practical realities of this and the tools required in order to meet those agreed times. That might apply for pre- or post-match workflows but might also be attributed towards live analysis too. During the game coach intervention is particularly relevant, given that it can directly impact player/team performance. Thus, the immediate feedback provided by coaches during the game should contain the most appropriate information that can help players/team to improve their performance, perhaps with the aid of analysis. That support might be helping to provide objective facts to any 'gut' feelings which either support or challenge those initial predisposed feelings. So, analysts must agree in advance sensible workflows for the focus in game, but also the communication methods, times of interruption and technologies needed to enable this objectivity to come into coach delivery in real time.

As each phase of the cycle develops, the focus will change and so the analyst must consider their role within each phase. Fundamentally, each piece of analysis that is to be completed must have a specific and measurable question to be answered. A *general* analysis should never be completed given that this is too vague and wide ranging, instead practitioners should in conjunction with coaches settle upon a number of core performance questions to answer, and then go about completing those with their knowledge. They must also consider the tools that they need to complete the job and invest wisely in technology and personnel if that is appropriate. Analysts may find themselves working in multiple cycles at different stages at once, perhaps completing the post-match from one game, whilst developing the pre-match for the next many weeks in advance, not to mention long-term profiling. This requires an awareness of professional self and a micropolitical literacy to manage expectation, time and output. Being able to help answer these performance questions requires an intricate level of understanding with analysts needing to spend time getting to better appreciate the coach and their coaching philosophy. An impactful coaching philosophy, not to be confused with playing philosophy, can help the analyst understand the underpinning pedagogical principles and values instilled to help answer performance questions, whilst for the coach, analysis data and output can help drive evolving coaching delivery mechanisms, values and attainments with the aid of a critical friend. Developing knowledge too of the game plan and the technical and tactical preferences is core, allowing the analyst to deeply understand play to better deliver insights, perhaps achieved through spending quality time with coaches and players, alongside a level of humility to being an ongoing student of the game. Ultimately, do you as an analyst understand what you are talking about deeply enough to still deliver even if your presentation got deleted?

Indeed, understanding people and process alongside deep sport knowledge are critical skills within the coaching process that all practitioners must develop. Such is the focus on a wide ranging and diverse interdisciplinary sports science team, analysts need to understand their role within that team, and how they might collaborate with others for success. That brings complexities, not least in the volume of data and conversation that will arise, and so maintaining the core analysis question at the heart, with developing communication skills is pivotal. To resolve performance questions a wider multi-faceted approach is key, finding the right balance, for the right impact, to the right group. It would appear with increasing relevance that a greater understanding of the role of the coach and the role of the analyst being key to support this inter-disciplinary approach is vital. The analyst is a crucial part of this, with Sarmento et al. (2015) discussing developing the team by having a dedicated performance analyst to help drive practice, further underpinned by the studies that highlighted that the coach-analyst relationship is crucial to the coaching process (Cushion, 2007; Wright et al., 2012, 2013). So, analysts must take time to understand their role, the people around them and building relationships with the coach to critically understand the plan.

Having done so, analysts need to develop ways in which to effectively deliver feedback into the coaching process by landing the message with the end user, at the appropriate time. They'll need to understand and utilise contemporary technology for this, whilst also developing an appreciation of pedagogical principles and underpinnings of feedback methods and strategies, individualising and adapting where necessary. Delivery should be short, sharp and concise, especially given that in live situations there may be just a short few seconds to deliver a message. Language is critical too, with analysts needing to utilise (or perhaps promote the use of) common language and definitions of phrases. All too often acronyms or colloquial-based interpretations become second nature to some, with tactical words or phrases utilised with increasing frequency, but not all will know these definitions and details of what is being discussed, leaving some in the dark, unwilling to put their reputation on the line for fear of not knowing. Common language definitions in personalised team dictionaries may be a way forwards to ensure commonality in language, with analysts being encouraged to promote and perhaps lead this.

Finally, analysts need to appreciate and know their role in the *so what?* conversations that will occur. Developing an understanding of how to take knowledge from each phase of the coaching process cycle to the next for impactful decision making is vital. That information might be performance analysis data that helps frame game conditioned responses and training design, or it might be helping set what it takes to win models and target setting from objective data analysis. Understanding the role that analysis has in training design, selection, recruitment or talent ID are all critical to role development and professional literacy. All of these will have to be considered in line with evolving constraints and learning environment considerations including the contextual, physical and cultural traits that affect how learning takes place. And in closing, analysts must also know their place, where in the coaching process cycle they are, which part of it do they fit into and does their message fit at all in the complex and messy reality that is coaching.

Concluding Remarks

So, readers need not worry that they've picked the wrong book up, but instead take away an increased appreciation of the complexities involved in coaching and the coaching process, understanding that their role is not undertaken in silo, void of context, influence or environment. This learning leads us to a better understanding of the close relationship between two messy and socially derived disciplines that we operate within. Coaching, like performance analysis, demands careful thought and a readiness to respond to the unexpected needing quick thinking, innovation and technology to drive practice and land messages with the ultimate end users. Learning how to fully navigate successfully through these uncertainties can be tricky, not least since there is so much uncertainty and many contextual factors that impact the journey. But the chapters in this book are designed to do just that, in a practical guide to the many evolving and dynamic interactive considerations and features of our exciting discipline.

References

Abraham, A., & Collins, D. (2011). Taking the next step: Ways forward for coaching science. *Quest, 63*(4), 366–384.

Bampouras, M., Cronin, C., & Miller, P. (2012). Performance analytic processes in elite sport practice: An exploratory investigation of the perspectives of a sport scientist, coach and athlete. *International Journal of Performance Analysis in Sport, 12*(2), 468–483.

Borrie, A., & Knowles, Z. (2003). Coaching science and soccer. In T. Reilly & A.M. Williams (Eds.), *Science and soccer* (pp. 187–198). London: Routledge.

Butterworth, A., O'Donoghue, P., & Cropley, B. (2013). Performance profiling in sports coaching: A review. *International Journal of Performance Analysis in Sport, 13*(3), 572–593.

Butterworth, A., Turner, D., & Johnstone, J. (2012). Coaches' perceptions of the potential use of performance analysis in badminton. *International Journal of Performance Analysis in Sport, 12*(2), 452–467.

Carling, C., Williams, A., & Reilly, T. (2005). *The handbook of soccer match analysis.* London: Routledge.

Cote, J., Salema, J., Trudel, P., Baria, A., & Russell, S. (1995). The coaching model: A grounded assessment of expert gymnastics coaches' knowledge. *Journal of Sport and Exercise Psychology, 17*(1), 1–17.

Cushion, C. J., Armour, K. M., & Jones, R. L. (2003). Coach education and continuing professional development: Experience and learning to coach. *Quest, 55*, 215–230.

Cushion, C. (2007). Modelling the complexity of the coaching process. *International Journal of Sports Science & Coaching, 2*(4), 395–401.

Cushion, C., Armour, K., & Jones, R. (2006). Locating the coaching process in practice: Models 'for' and 'of' coaching. *Physical Education and sport pedagogy, 11*(1), 83–99.

Cushion, C., & Lyle, J. (2010). Conceptual development in sports coaching. In J. Lyle & C. Cushion (Eds.), *Sports coaching: Professionalisation and practice* (pp. 1–14). London: Elsevier.

Cross, N. (1995). Coaching effectiveness in hockey: A Scottish perspective. *Scottish Journal of Physical Education, 23*(1), 27–39.

Dancs, H., & Kovacs, K. (2019). Project management issues in performance analysis. In M. Hughes, I.M. Franks, & H. Dancs (Eds.), *Essentials of performance analysis in sport* (pp. 21–31). London: Routledge.

D'Arripe-Longueville, F., Fournier, J.F., & Dubois, A. (1998). The perceived effectiveness of interactions between expert French Judo coaches and elite female athletes. *The Sport Psychologist, 12*, 317–332.

Duckett, J. (2012). *Objectivity in analysis: Performance analysis of football.* The Football Association. Retrieved from http://www.thefa.com/st-georges-park/discover/coaching/licensed -coaches-club/

Fairs, J.R. (1987). The coaching process: The essence of coaching. *Sports Coach, 11*(1), 17–19.

Fernandez-Echeverria, C., Mesquita, I., Conjero, M., & Perla Moreno, M. (2019). Perceptions of elite volleyball players on the importance of match analysis during the training process. *International Journal of Performance Analysis in Sport, 19*(2), 1–16.

Francis, J., & Jones, G. (2014). Elite rugby union players perceptions of performance analysis. *International Journal of Performance Analysis in Sport, 14*(1), 188–207.

Franks, I.M., Goodman, D., & Miller, G. (1983) Analysis of performance: Qualitative or quantitative? *Science Periodical of Research and Technology in Sport*, March, 1–8.

Gilbert, W., & Trudel, P. (2001). Learning to coach through experience: Reflection in model youth sport coaches. *Journal of Teaching in Physical Education, 21*, 16–34.

Groom, R., Cushion, C., & Nelson, L. (2011). The delivery of video-based performance analysis by England youth soccer coaches: Towards a grounded theory. *Journal of Applied Sports Psychology, 23*(1), 16–32.

Gutiérrez-Aguilar, Ó., Montoya-Fernández, M., Fernández-Romero, J.J., & Saavedra-García, A.M. (2016). Analysis of time-out use in handball and its influence on the game performance. *International Journal of Performance Analysis in Sport, 16*(1), 1–11.

Horne, S. (2013). The role of performance analysis in elite netball competition structures. In D.M. Peters & P. O'Donoghue (Eds.), *Performance analysis of sport IX* (pp. 30–37). London: Routledge.

Hughes, M., & Bartlett, R. (2008). What is performance analysis? In M. Hughes & I.M. Franks (Eds.), *The essentials of performance analysis: An introduction* (pp. 8–20). London: Routledge.

Jones, R. L., Armour, K. M., & Potrac, P. (2004). *Sports coaching cultures: From practice to theory.* London: Routledge.

Jones, R.L., & Wallace, M. (2005). Another bad day at the training ground: Coping with ambiguity in the coaching context. *Sport Education and Society, 10*(1), 119–134.

Kraak, W., Magwa, Z., & Terblanche, E. (2018). Analysis of South African semi-elite rugby head coaches' engagement with performance analysis. *International Journal of Performance Analysis in Sport, 18*(2), 350–366.

Knudson, V., & Morrison, S. (2002). *Qualitative analysis of human movement.* Champaign, IL: Human Kinetics.

Lyle, J. (1999). Coaching philosophy and coaching behaviour. In N. Cross & J. Lyle (Eds.), *The coaching process: Principles and practice for sport* (pp. 25–46). Oxford: Butterworth-Heinemann.

Lyle, J. (2002). *Sports coaching concepts.* London: Routledge.

MacKenzie, R., & Cushion, C. (2013). Performance analysis in football: A critical review and implications for future research. *Journal of Sport Sciences, 31*(6), 639–676.

MacLean, J.C., & Chelladurai, P. (1995). Dimensions of coaching performance: Development of a scale. *Journal of Sport Management, 9*, 194–207.

Martin, D., O'Donoghue, P., Bradley, J., & McGrath, D. (2021). Developing a framework for professional practice in applied performance analysis. *International Journal of Performance Analysis in Sport, 21*(6), 845–888.

Mayes, A., O'Donoghue, P.G., Garland, J., & Davidson, A. (2009). *The use of performance analysis and internet video streaming during elite netball preparation.* Poster presented at the 3rd international workshop of the international society of performance analysis of sport, Lincoln, UK, April.

Miles, A. (2003). *What is sports coaching?* Coachwise 1st4sport.

Nelson, L., & Groom, R. (2012). The analysis of athletic performance: Some practical and philosophical considerations, *Sport, Education and Society, 17*(5), 687–670.

O'Donoghue, P., & Mayes, A. (2013). Performance analysis, feedback & communication in coaching. In T. McGarry, P. O'Donghue, & J. Sampaio (Eds.), *Routledge handbook of sports performance analysis* (pp. 155–165). London: Routledge.

Painczyk, H., Hendricks, S., & Kraak, W. (2018). Intra and inter-reliability testing of a South African developed computerized notational system among Western Province Club Rugby. *International Journal of Sport Science Coaching, 13*(6), 1163–1170.

Sarmento, H., Bradley, P.S., & Travassos, B. (2015). The transition from match analysis to intervention: Optimizing the coaching process in elite futsal. *International Journal of Performance Analysis in Sport, 15*(2), 471–488.

Saury, J., & Durand, M. (1998). Practical knowledge in expert coaches: on-site study of coaching in sailing. *Research Quarterly in Exercise and Sport, 69*(3), 254–266.

Sherman, C., Crassini, B., Maschette, W., & Sands, R. (1997). Instructional sports psychology: A reconceptualisation of sports coaching as instruction. *International Journal of Sports Psychology, 28*(2), 103–125.

Thelwell, K. (2005). Foreword. In C. Carling, A.M. Williams, & T. Reilly (Eds.), *Handbook of soccer match analysis: A systematic approach to improving performance* (p. XVII). London, UK: Routledge.

Wright, C., Atkins, S., & Jones, B. (2012). An analysis of elite coaches' engagement with performance analysis services (match, notational analysis and technique analysis). *International Journal of Performance Analysis in Sport, 12*, 436–451.

Wright, C., Atkins, S., Jones, B., & Todd, J. (2013). The role of performance analysts within the coaching process: Performance Analysts Survey 'The role of performance analysts in elite football club settings.' *International Journal of Performance Analysis in Sport, 13*(1), 240–261.

Wright, C., Carling, C., & Collins, D. (2014). The wider context of performance analysis and it application in the football coaching process. *International Journal of Performance Analysis in Sport, 14*(3), 709–733.

Wright, C., Carling, C., Lawlor, C., & Collins, D. (2016). Elite football player's engagement with performance analysis. *International Journal of Performance Analysis in Sport, 16*(1), 1007–1032.

2

EMERGING TECHNOLOGY AND INTERACTIVE FEEDBACK

Andrew Butterworth

Introduction

Innovation and advancement in technologies continue to rise on an industrial scale, with an incredible influx of new, fast and efficient systems able to seemingly streamline our everyday lives. In sport, and indeed performance analysis, the influx is just as widespread, so much so that technology is claimed to be the most important factor driving the competitiveness of the sport industry (Ratten, 2020). Specifically, the use of technology is being used more and more in order to facilitate performance improvements, with sport and science sharing the same goal of transcending limits, innovating and progressing (Trabal, 2013). In some quarters, the sport industry is labelled as the most technologically innovated, driven by a desire for constant improvement, creativity and innovation in practice (Riot & James, 2013). This has subsequently changed the fundamental role of the analyst, with automation freeing more time for *actual analysis* to be completed rather than being used for laborious data collection.

Of all the sport sciences, performance analysis is the discipline which leans most heavily on this emerging technology, utilising the developing equipment to provide more streamlined and efficient learning opportunities. In doing so, as part of the dynamic and evolving coaching process, performance analysis seeks to identify areas of tactical or technical interest and enhance the quality of interactive feedback provided. This enhanced quality allows more efficient communication back to coaches and players as part of the ongoing feedback loop.

Feedback and Technology

If athletes are to make improvements, then they require feedback as an essential tool in their armoury. Task intrinsic feedback from senses provides athletes with

DOI: 10.4324/9781003226659-2

immediate responses from sight, sound, tactile and proprioceptive sources, whilst augmented external information can be provided by many sources including subjectively from coaches or peers, or more objectively using performance analysis and technology. For coaches too, technology can help them in their role, with Franks and Miller's (1986) research citing that coaches recall around 45% of events from a match, a similar number to that of Laird and Waters (2008) who found 59% in their repeat study. Whilst there remains some debate around the accuracy of these numbers and the contextual factors that might influence them, what is clear is that there is a significant proportion of matches (and presumably training too) currently, which are destined to be forgotten. That is unless performance analysis, using technology, helps to plug that gap, filling in parts of the information deficit and in turn providing a more valid and reliable recall of performance. Sophisticated outputs have now gained enough functionality and traction to do this in near real time with increasingly quick feedback available which holds promise for enhancing learning.

Technological innovation is indeed now core for the majority of sports teams, more specifically within the sport science and performance analysis teams, and whilst its importance is not new, streamlining efficiencies and expanding capabilities are. Rethinking or reapplying ideas and workflows in a different manner using such technologies has the potential to significantly benefit the end user. Largely, most of these developments have come in line with huge increases in computer power, and a flood of contemporary and emergent technology companies keen to impress a more streamlined experience (Hutchins & Rowe, 2013). The use of smartphones has driven change too; you'd be hard pressed to find a single athlete, coach or analyst in the professional industry now without one by their side for the majority of their day. Smartphones have changed the way that we live our everyday lives, but also in how we capture, analyse and deliver feedback, providing analysis in a quicker more convenient manner, whilst enhanced user experiences on these devices have allowed for this to become more comfortable. Of course, there are many other drivers of change in the industry too (e.g. generational preferences), and phones are just one, but what is clear is that often sport technology innovations are invented first elsewhere, before translating to use in our environments after careful developments and testing procedures (Ratten, 2020).

Ultimately learning is the key driver and an intended outcome for the role of a performance analyst, and the same also applies when we consider the intended outcome of new technologies being adopted. Zeimers et al. (2019) describe organisational learning as a process through which organisations learn about interactions with internal and external environments. Therefore, for analysts, if we learn and adapt from these technologies, we might bring about a change in practice, translating knowledge and insight to our players in a more meaningful manner so that they can positively impact the outcome of performance. Knowledge will likely have been formed from numerous iterations of these technologies drawing upon multiple sources, and so the integration of those together is critical for success, otherwise we might see a very disparate and messy outcome. If successful, this coherent messaging will hopefully bring about better results, suggesting that to continue moving forwards knowledge must be derived and combined from a range of technologies, rather than each working in silo.

It isn't all one way though, with some sports organisations or specific persons reluctant to adopt technology, citing a desire to maintain current practices (Mallen, 2019), or a perceived threat to the role or diminished responsibilities (Butterworth et al., 2012). This is far from the intention, with the role of the coach, analyst and player remaining critical in the process, providing tacit knowledge through experience, which machines will never be able to. Cabrillo and Dahms (2018) discuss this, referring to the concept of intellectual capital, that is the intangible knowledge-based resources that include humans and relationships. A human's experience, skill and ability in their sport is a way of involving vital intuition in the decision-making process enabling final decisions to be made on technologically driven facts, but also on feelings. Technology should never take over entirely, it is simply not smart enough and not human enough, if we were ever to allow that then sport would be a much poorer product, with increasing levels of predictability achieved by stifling creativity.

In that vein, research in Swedish elite football highlights a number of challenges and problems with the implementation of performance analysis technologies (Barker-Ruchti et al., 2021). This, and various other studies have sought to consider the impact of technologies within the coaching process, with no clear consensus showing a positive linear relationship. Whilst some technologies have been shown to enhance relationships, training behaviours and safety, research evidence underpinned by pedagogical principles and a sound conceptual base to support their practice is lacking. Further barriers to the use of technology in sport come through the astronomical pricing of some of the latest products. Whilst for some money is not an issue, it is a real issue to sports receiving less funding, without feeling left behind. Barker-Ruchti et al. (2021) refer to this as a digital divide, enhancing inequalities across different settings e.g. women's sport (Ericsson & Horgby, 2020) and heightening pressures to invest. These are real concerns and ones that should not go un-reported, with Chapter 10 of this book discussing financial implications and solutions in more detail.

The Old Days

When Charles Reep began his analysis at half time of Bristol Rovers 1-0 loss to Swindon Town in 1950, he recorded 147 attacking plays in the second half by the Wiltshire based side, doing so with pencil and paper. There was no video, no hardware and no software. It wasn't until 1983 that Sony released the first consumer camcorder, the Betamovie BMC-100P which had a number of features, though most of them were manual including the zoom, white balance, exposure and focus. This was soon replaced by the more commonly known Betamax, though that too was quickly trumped by the introduction of JVC's VHS format which became the choice for many amateur film makers, and early performance analysis practitioners. Other technologies tried to emulate or success the VHS, with video compact cassettes trying before the take-off of DVDs in the early 2000s. HD DVD followed later in the decade at a similar time to which performance analysis was gaining significant popularity.

As cameras developed, the ability to capture more efficiently evolved, which was usually then issued out post-match using DVD burners, the bulky stacked devices to share and distribute video from games was commonplace for a period of time, with users needing a certain level of knowledge, to work out what +R and −R formatted discs actually were, and save considerable cursing, having spent hours burning on the wrong format or having purchased the wrong disc type. With the advent of more powerful computers and Apple Mac becoming the machine of choice, the ability to capture directly into a computer evolved, with the Canopus box an early mainstay to facilitate this. Using firewire connections, this somewhat temperamental video conversion device effectively played its part (most of the time) and allowed analysts to revolutionise analysis workflows by providing early opportunities for feedback during the match. BlackMagic boxes and more recently AJA U-Tap devices have since streamlined the video capture process immeasurably and provided a more reliable source.

Alongside these hardware developments, software was emerging too. Early mainstays in the late 1990s included ProZone which was revolutionary in its day using an eight-camera system to track each football players movement multiple times per second. Soon performance analysis coding software began to appear on the market with Dartfish and the then named Sportstec early players in this field. As time and technology grew on, the specificity and power of analysis tools has grown immeasurably. Now, there are a seemingly bewildering number of new and emerging technologies available to analysts, in a growing market with innovation at an all-time high. More and more companies evolve and seek to provide the best products possible, providing some welcome competition for a market which was once dominated by just a select handful. This chapter seeks to provide an overview of some of those technologies, unearthing the significant capabilities and possibilities that they bring, helping to align together and bring understanding of what might be suitable for a particular given environment. The content does not seek to endorse any particular product or recommend which should be used, especially given that each environment and context has different needs. Instead, this work cuts through the marketing strategies to provide a balanced enquiry into this exciting, dynamic and evolving market.

Hardware

Computer hardware was invented to 'compute' and solve problems, whilst also storing and retrieving data alongside the management of communications and the manipulation of multimedia. Buried deep inside each hardware is a complex web of interconnecting circuits that transform signals into useable outputs in our digital age, and whilst most of us rarely see or comprehend this complexity, it is that web which allows us as performance analysts, to draw heavily on in our job role. Now, there are a wide number of devices available on the market which we'll examine here in turn, each providing a potential benefit in our workflows.

Handheld Cameras

The advent of the consumer camcorder in 1983 paved the way for much of the video analysis work we see today, with early machines able to record snippets of training or matches for review in a post-event manner, using largely manual processes. Now, the speed of camera hardware is such that near instant replay is available and the processes are inherently streamlined. Innovation saw the fast rise of camera technology and in the early 2000s, high-definition cameras came more widely to the market, offering a better clarity of image and enhanced visual for the end user. For many years, such cameras were the mainstay of the majority of analysts, a key part of their toolkit as they manually captured their sport taking their trusty devices with them wherever they went. Sony, Panasonic and Canon cameras have been consistently at the forefront of this market, with popular models such as the Sony HVR-A1E, the Panasonic HC series and Canon Legria HFG40 all widely used.

For some, especially those on lower budgets, HD cameras remain, though for many 4K cameras, promising even higher quality and enhanced recognition started to take over, with the same manufacturers again dominating the market. Offering four times the definition of HD, these cameras are powerful, though of course with that power and image quality, they inherently produce larger file sizes and price tags. Further problems are also sometimes found in the capture process, as capture conversion boxes such as the BlackMagic and AJA U-Tap not always being able to process at the same high quality, with the end product in the software programme of choice not always remaining at full 4K quality. 5K, 6K and now even 8K cameras are all in production, but again have some of the same problems and so their use, for now at least, remains largely in the professional film and media industries, having not yet fully transcended into our performance analysis sphere.

With all of these handheld cameras, the angle and vantage point have always been an area of considerable attention and sometimes concern. With many training or match environments not having a suitable vantage point to gain the all-important height, many have to invest in fixed or temporary gantries to allow analysts to capture the optimal angle. These structures largely do their job effectively, allowing for a wider angle and more players to be in shot. For the analyst though being at that greater height means being at the mercy of the weather even more (unless having the luxury of an indoor sport), and with some temporary gantries feeling more than a little unstable at times, there is perhaps nothing worse knowing that you have to clamber up the scaffolding when a blustery Sunday morning is forecast. In response, there are now a number of

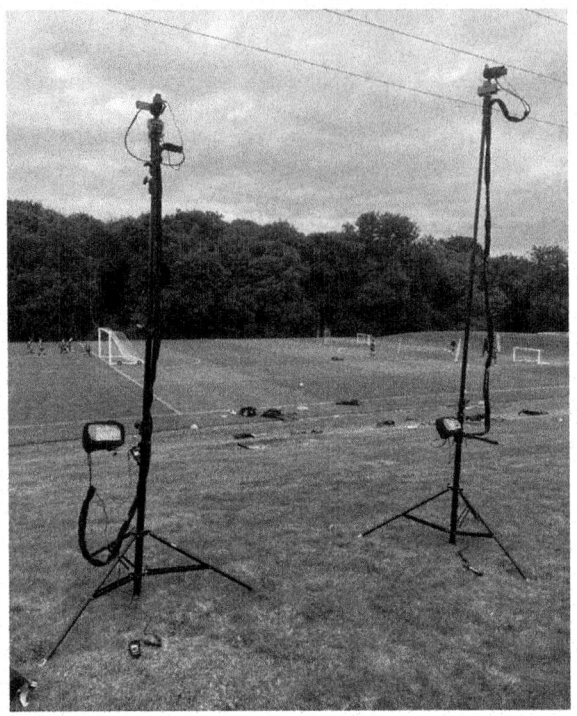

FIGURE 2.1 Hi-Pods.

hi-pod offerings, a retractable device which winches the camera securely into the air, whilst maintaining the ability to control the camera at ground level (Figure 2.1). Contemporary designs of hi-pods now are lighter, more stable and easier to manoeuvre.

NacSport's AP Capture system offers a portable mast system which is a 4K-quality camera operated by a physical joystick or a joystick app, and is captured locally onto a hardware device. The system also offers up opportunity to live stream at the same time which may offer some a revenue option or exposure and awareness options. HI-POD and EVS EndZone offer other options in portable towers, with similar functionality attached to each.

Drones

In further developing the angles and heights possible, drones are now a popular tool, providing a bird's eye tactical view of performance. These devices offer the capture of virtually every angle, bar those occupied by trees, with unprecedented access to heights never seen before by any other device (Figure 2.2). Rather than being restricted by stationary cameras, drones can be swiftly moved to offer the most suitable angle for capture. Live feed outputs can be obtained, opening up live coding and feedback opportunities with the technology. Though, the main

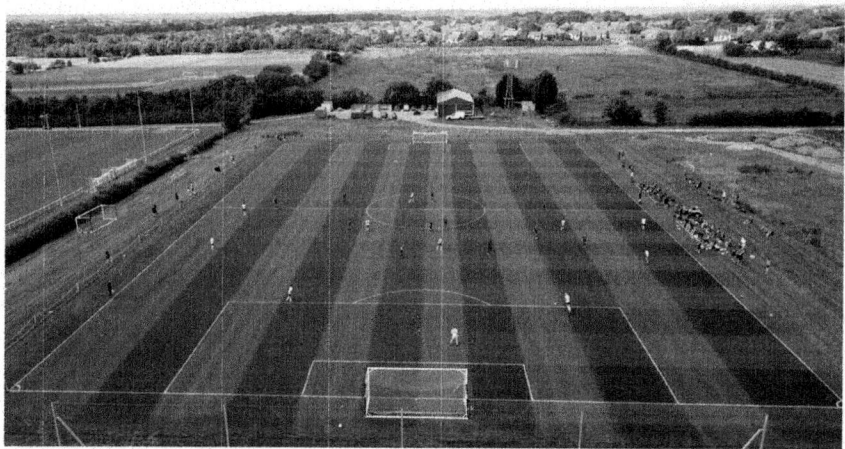

FIGURE 2.2 Drone footage.

drawback at present is the battery life, with most only lasting for around 25 minutes and so when we consider the time to ascend and descend, this limits the actual amount of training or match play captured.

IP Cameras, AI and Automatic Tracking

For many, a permanent built in solution to capturing video is desired. IP cameras, an acronym for internet protocol cameras, use an internet network to record, share and send footage data. Generally, these cameras are more commonly used for surveillance purposes in the CCTV industry, though now, these devices are becoming commonplace in the performance analysis industry. Utilising the same technologies, IP cameras can be installed permanently at a venue with a feed out of the camera into the analysts capturing device always available. Pan, tilt, zoom (PTZ) cameras are the most common, and offer the analyst the opportunity to manually control the features of the camera using a joystick or app which responds in near real time. This capture of footage provides the optimal vantage point, with multiple IP cameras used by many to capture different angles of the same performance to enhance analysis processes.

Though highly popular, IP cameras still rely somewhat on a manual control of the device in order to capture all of the desired performance. To that end, the use of artificial intelligence (AI) technologies to help automatically capture the footage without the need for manual intervention is becoming commonplace. AI-enabled IP cameras think and learn about settings, boundaries and image processing through a quick recognition of what is a scene (e.g. the sport being played) and what is background. Sophisticated systems use complex algorithms to automatically blend multiple camera angles, zoom, focus and pan automatically to stitch together a capture of performance. In recent years there has been a significant shift towards AI-enabled tracking cameras, since they save the manual need to film and so free up the analyst to focus on other areas of their job. Now, analysts working in silo can code simultaneously without needing to worry about remembering to pan the camera as well, whilst others can elect to analyse more efficiently in real time safe in the knowledge that the AI is capturing every move. Springing up across multiple sports in training grounds and centres across the world, automated cameras are still somewhat in their infancy, but show signs of becoming the norm, in a new digitally driven and intelligent AI age.

Spiideo

Boldly, Spiideo claim that manually filming footage is a waste of time and money and that panoramic footage is essential for high-quality feedback, also stating that live video access can make the difference to match results. Their solution is a permanent camera solution installed at training grounds and playing venues, offering instant access to anything that happens in a time sensitive manner. Two camera systems are available, the detailed 4k Spiideo camera and the 4K ultra-wide Spiideo wide system to offer full-pitch stitching and panorama. The cameras are accessed by an app offered on Apple products, or via a computer on the internet which provides options to automatically view and upload footage with live and post event tagging also available in your preferred analysis capture programme.

Hudl Focus

Installed permanently in a training ground or venue, the Hudl Focus camera system offers an instant access capture device which can automatically record training and fixtures. Capturing up to four angles simultaneously, including 180-degree panoramic, as well as automated AI-enabled tracking technology, the camera system provides HD video output as well as a handy scoreboard inlay feed. Accessed via an App for Apple or Android (Figure 2.3), the system also offers an integrated Hudl.com upload feature and an IP capture solution live into Hudl SportsCode. A portable version is now on the way too, with Hudl Flex soon to come to market offering a solution for multiple venues from a single device.

GameOn

The premium brand and technologically driven GameOn Technologies system delivers a high-end solution for the capture of video in real time. Using extensive high-quality camera products installed in permanent fixed positions, cameras are operated from an app with automatic tracking once the recording starts. Once being captured, the associated video player app designed for Apple mobile devices allows for live replaying as capture takes place (opening up live video to the

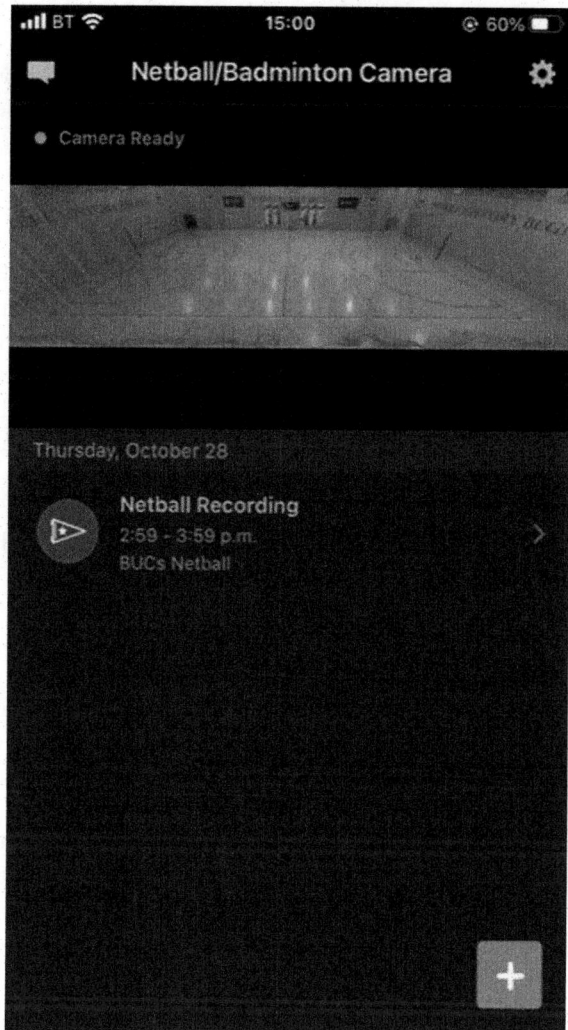

FIGURE 2.3   Hudl focus mobile application.

bench), basic telestration, amongst a host of control zoom and switching features. The system is also compatible with coding software to allow for live capture and coding by the analyst in the stands.

VEO

The AI-enabled VEO camera is a portable solution which can live stream matches externally and offers a live capture solution back to a coding software of choice too. The camera is lightweight and portable meaning that unlike many other systems, it can be used by teams travelling away from home if the correct vantage point can be sought. Uploaded automatically to their web-based server VEO Editor, the system can also automatically tag a very small number of events using AI and will also, using the same AI, track players through the captured video. Subsequently this leads to the automatic creation of heat maps, interactive 2D maps and match graphics including momentum.

Provispo

With a range of solutions, Provispo are offering a flexible approach to IP solutions in capturing video footage. Their fixed SportsCam Automatic combines two 4K cameras to record full pitches in panoramic view, tactical and broadcast with AI recording and tracking according to the players and ball. SportsCam Control meanwhile is a joystick-operated device which is manually controlled and able to be used as a fixed or mobile solution, the SportsCam Goal meanwhile is a fixed solution which uses AI to track the play on half of a pitch with inbuilt pan, tilt and zoom. All solutions feedback via the Recorder which allows for scheduling of events and a real-time wireless ingestion of the feeds for storage and analysis.

RedZone

Seeking to professionalise the delivery of hardware technology infrastructure in high performance sport, RedZone offers high-end solutions to AI-enabled capture technology. The company offer an array of camera systems with associated cabling, switches and poles to training ground and stadiums. There is also a mobile offer for away games and the opportunity to engage in live feedback and video replay by innovative means including big screens attached to golf carts. They offer a bespoke design and build service to tailor needs to the end user, though these services naturally come at a cost which will be prohibitive to many.

Network Infrastructure

Regardless of which camera system, ingesting multiple video feeds and collaborative coding on multiple devices is now commonplace in high-end performance analysis workflows. A growing majority of analysis departments at the highest end will seek to intake a number of video angles at a time, allowing for reviews to be completed from different views for a deeper analysis. Additional coding needs from coaches in real time also mean that software mentioned later in this chapter allow for multiple analysts to code collaboratively on a single timeline for faster and wider reviews. Widely used in many sports, rugby union perhaps leads the way here, with the coach commonly found at games with the analysts, reviewing coding and footage in real time. For both of these set ups to be successful, knowledge of networking set up and equipment is vital, to ensure that the feeds and coding can be set up effectively.

Comprising two or more computers connected either wirelessly or by physical wires, a network allows the transmission, exchange or sharing of data. Each network is bespoke, built to serve the needs of the end user with specific hardware and software. Hardware required will vary, but fundamentals include routers, switches and specification cabling to enable machines to communicate with each other. The vast majority of network needs for performance analysis systems will work as either a local area network (LAN) or wireless local area network (WLAN), allowing them to connect over relatively short distances to transmit video and data via a coding platform of choice. Hardwired LAN networks offer better reliability, however require sometimes extensive and impractical cabling to and from gantries, hence wireless WLAN options are popular, though prone to drop out. For the analyst, taking time to learn the technical needs and inner workings of networks is increasingly important, especially given the growing prominence of real time systems for live analysis delivery.

Once enabled, these networks can help to provide bench-side video and data on hardware devices. Given the technological advances and speed at which feedback can be provided, there has now been a shift towards coaches seeking to have video and data available to them as matches and training progress. For data, this largely means the sharing of output windows which, as described later in this chapter, offer data linked to analysts coding in real time presented in graphical format. As games progress the output windows update with the latest numbers from the game, allowing more objective and informed decisions to be made. These output windows are typically sent via wireless infrastructure such as NetGear or Ruckus routers, sometimes with the aid of signal boosters such as Mikrotik cubes, to tablet devices to allow decisions to be made with the aid of data. Furthermore, there is also a shift towards additional information to coaches in real time with video now a popular tool to allow for instantaneous feedback. Training environments now see big screens and portable projectors pitch side using this networking capability to allow for drills to be replayed and discussed, stimulating conversation and action (Figure 2.4).

Fast becoming a tool that some coaches find useful to their practice, the evolution of live feedback is expanding, especially where rules in individual sports allow and permit the use of technology on the bench. Such is the desire for video, technology has responded with many solutions now available via tablet devices to allow for video and data to be streamed down in near real time, adding objectivity to decision making in pressurised situations (Figure 2.5). The following are software that sit on advanced tablet hardware, but fit well for discussion into the current section here as a natural follow on, having already discussed networking.

Hudl Replay

Using Apple iPad technologies and a bespoke software platform, Hudl Replay (Figure 2.6) offers a near instantaneous replay of critical events within a match or training session to coaches on the bench. Collaboration between devices,

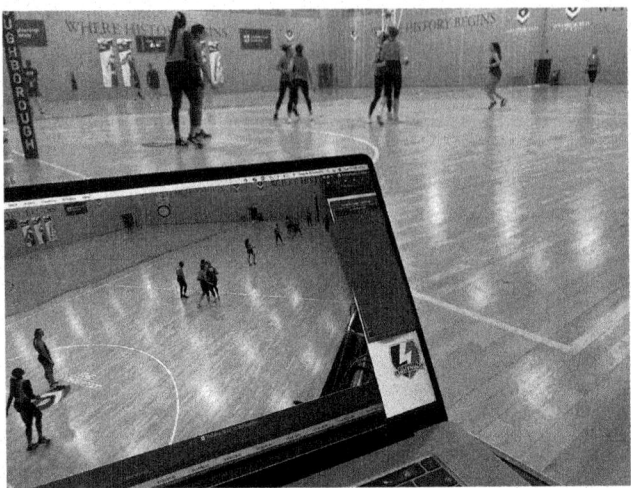

FIGURE 2.4 Live replay in training.

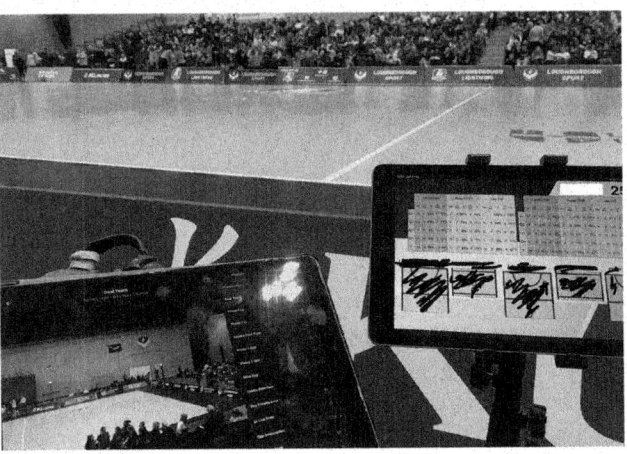

FIGURE 2.5 Live video and data in match.

including the analysts main capture machine, ensures that everything is mirrored on the iPad device, allowing for decisions to be made having reviewed the video and data first.

Catapult Pro Video – Focus (Tablet Based)

Now owned by Catapult, Focus is a product on tablet devices, primarily iPads. Using a networked router through either wired or wireless means, the product allows users to review captured video alongside codes near instantly (Figure 2.7). The software also allows for collaborations and coding over multiple machines,

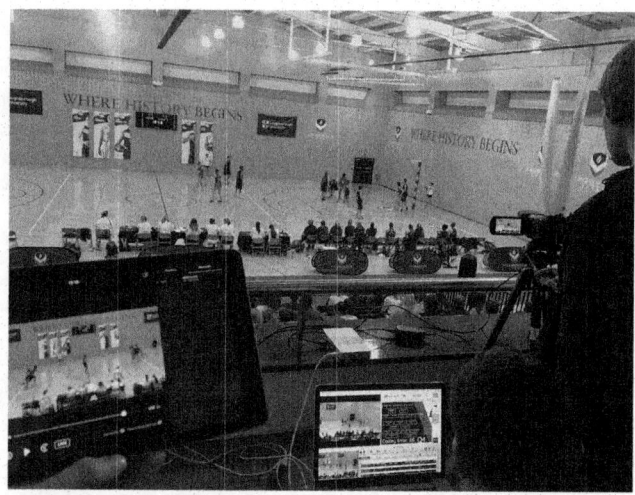

FIGURE 2.6 Hudl replay.

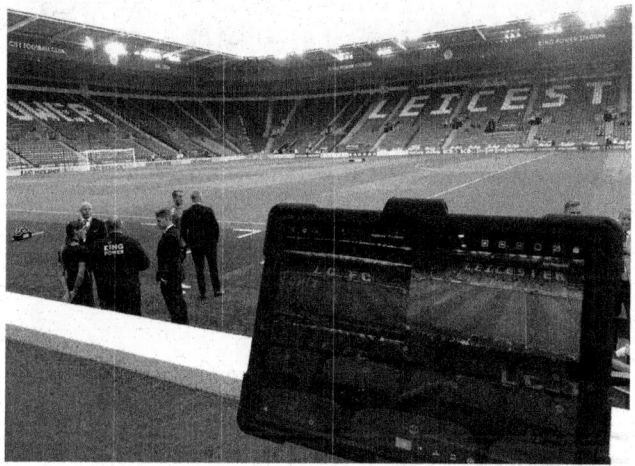

FIGURE 2.7 Catapult Pro Video – Focus, a multi-angle iPad application.

meaning pre-defined video clips can be built into organisers ready for presentation back to players and coaches. Archiving and sharing of built playlists enable further collaboration and speed of delivery over the networked infrastructure.

CoachStation

NacSport product CoachStation promises to help coaches make the right decisions by streaming images and data directly from another NacSport software program. Streamed live to the bench, the product seeks to deliver real-time data to where it is needed most, receiving images and data as soon as the capture is

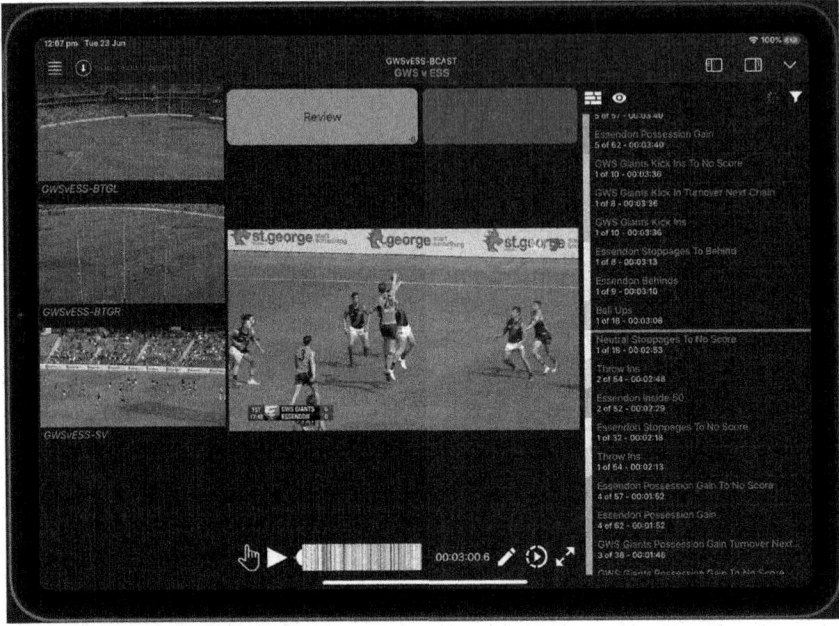

FIGURE 2.8 Piston.

started allowing replay, rewind and re-watch facilities. Data from coding can be displayed too in the form of a dashboard, delivering specific metrics to a specified device.

Piston

Based on iPads, Piston by Fulcrum Technologies seeks to accelerate learning moment during training and performances (Figure 2.8). Ingesting multiple feeds and then distributing in a single package using wireless infrastructure, it claims to enhance the knowledge transfer process and create real impact.

Virtual Reality

Some organisations and clubs are now investing in even more advanced learning methods by immersing their athletes in virtual reality (VR). VR uses bespoke designed headsets based upon gyroscopes and motion sensors which sense small movements in the body, head and hands of those wearing it. Small stereoscopic HD displays in the headset, coupled with fast and lightweight processors, provide an immersive reality. The technology is claimed by some researchers to overcome the limitations of video-based feedback, which they claim is restrictive, and allows immersive learning to foster a better learning experience (Bideau et al., 2010). VR creates a computer-generated environment which can deceive the brain and create a feeling of being present in the virtual space. The underlying principle behind VR is that by being immersed it provides realistic imagery and experience which gives participants the perception that it is real, thus forcing them to respond to the situation. This simulated environment can be set with specific tasks and problems which the athletes are asked to overcome, with some research indicating positive learning enhancements compared to typical imagery-based training (Bedir & Erhan, 2021).

Eye Tracking

More advanced still, the use of eye tracking technology has been used in some sporting contexts, including the sport of climbing. Helping with both athlete learning and extensively in coach education development, the technology characterises the underpinning cognitive-perceptual mechanisms that underpin expertise (Mitchell et al., 2020). Lightweight mobile eye tracking devices provide a precise and non-invasive measurement down to the millisecond of where, for how long and what visual attention is focussed on. Such data can help to pinpoint if perceptual gaze is in fact focussing on the most important cues in sport and if the individual involved can be retrained or educated as to which is focus on instead. Yet to be extensively rolled out across all sports, the use of eye tracking technology is set to grow in years to come.

Software

Until the late 1940s, the term *software* was relatively unknown with the early development infrequent at that time, becoming more embedded from 1950 onwards. At this time, computer hardware companies supplied software alongside hardware, built in to their early machines as applications programmes, though it was as recent as 1990 that commercial software became more readily available, offering reliable solutions at a more reasonable price. Initial Windows operating systems came in the early 1990s with Windows 1, 2, 3 and 3.1 (complete with minesweeper), the early systems. If born, readers will likely remember the Windows 95, which started a dynasty of more efficient, reliable and innovative software options. Powerful word and number processing software were placed on these which helped early analysts with the organisation of their data, and of course the highlight, Clippy. Meanwhile, Apple first released System 1 in 1984, a revolutionary operating system at its time with a graphical interface. Systems 1 through to 9 evolved rapidly bringing new features and better security until 2001, when Apple released its first Mac OS X operating system, which perhaps unknowingly at the time, signalled the start of Apple domination in the performance analysis sphere. Cheetah, the first OS X had many of the features still used today including the dock and photo-realistic icons. Many iterations of the OS X have followed, adding countless features and efficiencies, alongside enhanced user experiences.

As both Windows and Mac have provided their operating systems, the choice of hardware and so subsequently software became Apple and Mac OS X, due largely to increased processing power, memory and efficiency. And whilst the Windows suite of software has improved vastly, Mac remains the OS of choice for most in the industry. The once Windows exclusive software companies are now investing huge sums of money in translating their products into OS X languages, in an attempt to gain some of the popular market share.

Data Capture and Coding

The fundamental process of capturing video and coding for analysis purposes has remained largely unchanged, despite the increase in technologies available to help do this. However the video is ingested, a software is required in order to process that alongside data generated from third party sources, or from the analyst themselves coding. There are now a growing number of technologies in the sphere which analysts are able to select for their environment. The vast majority are sport blind, and so can be tailored for use in any sport.

Hudl SportsCode

The Mac based software Hudl SportsCode allows users to capture video and custom code events either as the game progresses, or post-event. Video can be ingested from multiple sources, either a single camera operated by the analyst, or multiple angles from IP or broadcast feeds simultaneously. Users create their own code windows, tailored to meet the needs of the coach and other end users before using these to capture the events as they happen in game. SportsCode uses a timeline feature which chronologically charts the events as they happen, syncing them automatically with the video to allow for an immediate review. Figure 2.9 is an example of multi-angle capture timeline. Using

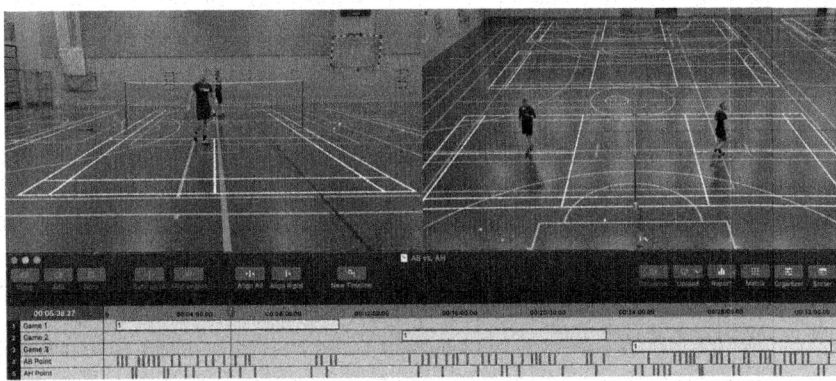

FIGURE 2.9 Hudl SportsCode multi-angle capture.

collaborative coding, analysts can set up numerous machines to be networked to each other, allowing a different code window to be used on each by different analysts, all running back to a master capture device. This capability opens up the opportunity for more live coding to be completed and for analysts to be given specific in-match roles to focus on (e.g. attack or defence) within their match day coding role.

The software allows users to analyse what matters to them in real time, reviewing mid-game where required in order to pass on information and help generate conversation. To facilitate this review process in game, SportsCode has an output window feature using scripting capabilities. These output windows produce graphical real-time reports which are fully customisable using scripting language and the design toolkit feature which provides a library of button, script and graph assets (Figure 2.10). Though the initial set up and scripting of the window can be a little time consuming, once built the reports are powerful and dynamic. Output windows can be customised to include data, graphics, charts and also be linked to immediate video review and sent to the coaches via tablet devices. Post-game, users are able to utilise these outputs to help deliver their debriefs, and will also make use of the databasing and movie organiser features. Databases offer the opportunity to combine coded instances from multiple matches to keep a longitudinal log of performances, whilst movie organisers allow for specific clips from a game to be selected ready for use in feeding back to coaches and players. More recent developments have seen the advent of their Insight product, which promises enhanced levels of integration and data analysis in real time from multiple sources.

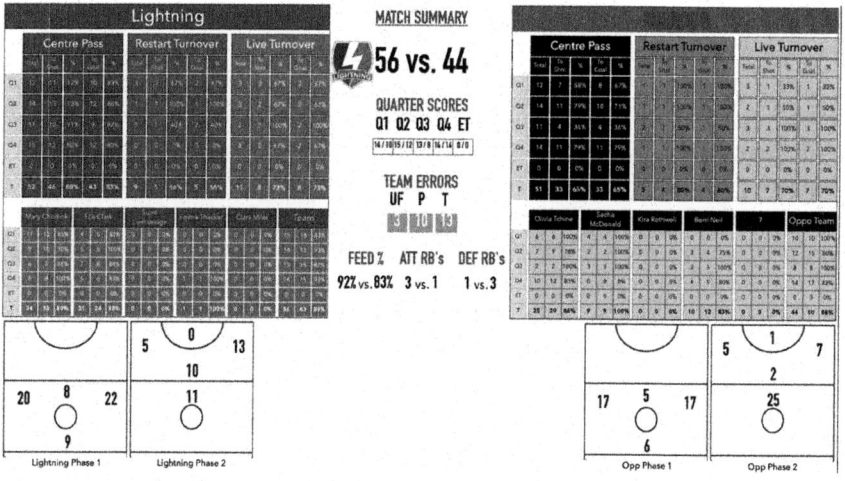

FIGURE 2.10 Hudl SportsCode output window.

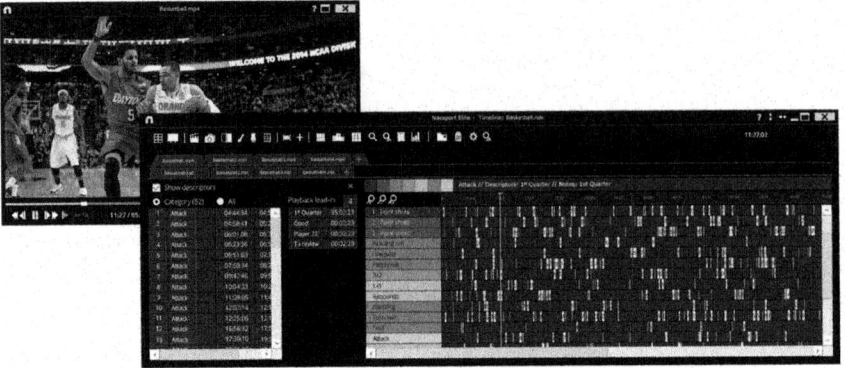

FIGURE 2.11 NacSport timeline.

NacSport

Available on Windows and now Mac, NacSport offers varying different levels of product, depending on the feature set users require. A basic read-only viewer product allows users to analyse tagged video, but not capture or tag themselves, which offers an entry level product to review analysis by others. As the product level increases, ingesting multiple video feeds is possible, using the earlier mentioned IP solutions and the RTSP box, or by single cameras too. Once in, the video can be tagged using custom built templates to get the data needed for the game at hand. As tagging is being completed either in game or post-game, the NacSport timeline updates, in chronological order with video associated with those tags for quick review (Figure 2.11). NacSport offers a dashboard feature which enables users to create impactful statistical outputs to display the data that they are generating. Elements of the dashboard are interactive, linked directly to the video and helps drive interactive feedback and can be delivered to coaches in near-real time.

In the more advanced versions of the software, a key feature is the graphic descriptor tool. This allows users to mark specific areas on their own pitch/court images in relation to the tagging they are completing and create heat maps for particular purposes (Figure 2.12). Additional useful tools in the software include the search feature which allows users to find specific tags or descriptors, giving the opportunity to find specific moments of interest. The presentation window meanwhile gives coaches and analysts the chance to filter clips from a timeline into lists that they can organise and use to present back in meetings.

Angles

Described as the next-generation performance data editor, Angles, built by Fulcrum Technologies, claims to present unique and powerful ways to work with

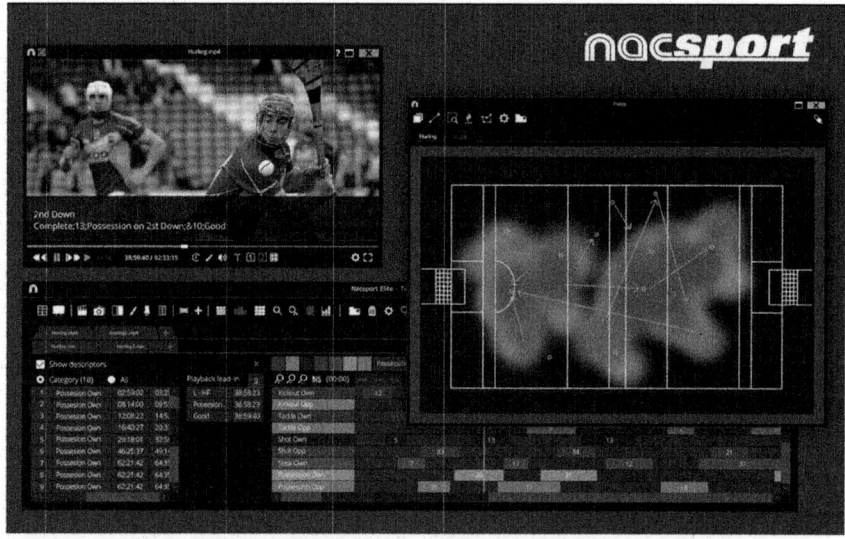

FIGURE 2.12 NacSport graphic descriptor tool.

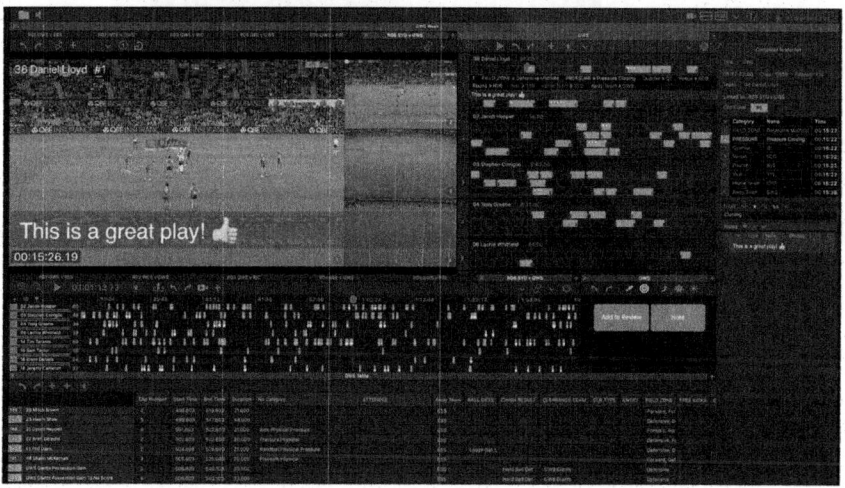

FIGURE 2.13 Angles.

data (Figure 2.13). Flexible and customisable the interface allows multiple views to capture live video from multiple angles alongside the ability to MarkUp (code) events during capture or post. Clips can be notated whilst presentations, filtering, archiving and file management are all offered as part of this emerging software. Data and movies are easily exported into other applications, whilst data can also be imported from other sources too if desired.

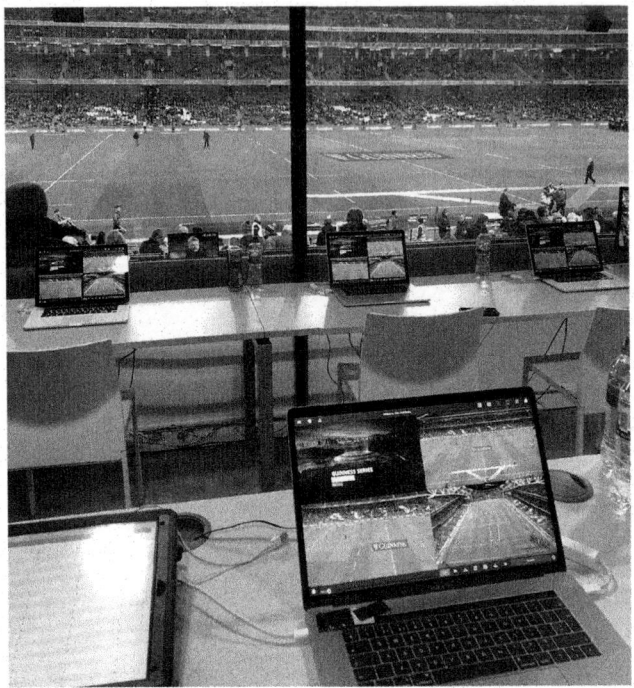

FIGURE 2.14 Catapult Pro Video – Focus, networked machines.

Catapult Pro Video – Focus (Computer Based)

The Windows and Mac-based Focus software allows analysts to record multiple angles simultaneously, alongside immediate tag and reviewing capabilities. Able to ingest multiple angles via either IP feeds or local cameras, the software seeks to allow information to be translated for practical implementation during coaching interventions. Multiple machines can be networked together to provide collaboration opportunities with input from analysts and coaches simultaneously whilst also working together to produce presentations for delivery at quarter or half times (Figure 2.14). Catapult also offers their popular MatchTracker product which ingests technical, tactical and physical data in real time to allow for the analysis of trends, tactics and opposition using multiple sources. With unlimited import capabilities, the software is an extremely powerful means by which to combine and visualise outputs for real impact and decision making (Figure 2.15).

Longomatch

Usable on both Mac and Windows alike, Longomatch offers an entry-level version of their software for free. This basic version allows users to gain the essentials of video analysis for no fee, providing them with limited video imports and analysis capabilities. The reasonably priced paid versions of the software increase in

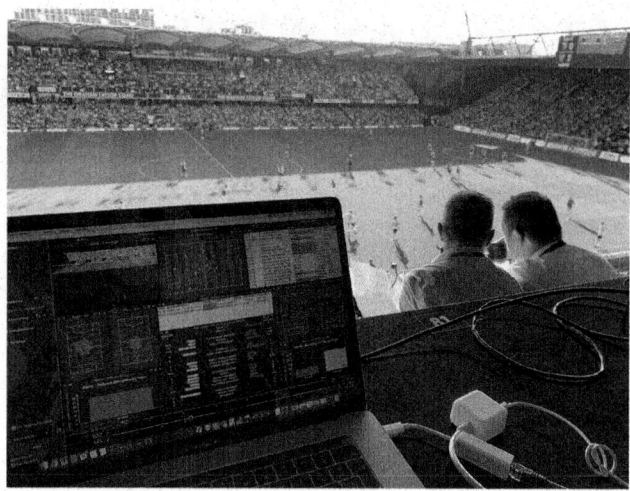

FIGURE 2.15 Catapult Pro Video – MatchTracker.

functionality and allow for multi capture, databasing, event tagging and import/ export to .xml files compatible for other software. The tool offers a viable option for those with little or no budget.

Kinovea

Entirely free, a Windows only based product, Kinovea offers a very basic video analysis package which is most suited to technique analysis. The software allows users to import videos in, before then exploring slow motion, annotations and drawing, notes and measurement of angles. There is also the option to live import video, though this is done with very basic webcam type devices and so the quality naturally suffers as a result. Highlighted for use in individual sports or analysing the technique of individuals in a team sport, Kinovea offers an entry level product for those with no budget.

Telestration

Telestration is the drawing of graphics and annotations over the top of existing pre-captured video sequences. Popularised initially through TV broadcasting, analysts now regularly use the technology to help illustrate key tactical and technical points of note in an attempt to enhance learning (Figure 2.16). Whilst most existing research in the field lies within medical literature, where it is used regularly as an aid to learning, seminal research from Jones et al. (2020) have also examined the worth of the tool specifically in sport using football as a case study. Their results indicated that telestration has an important role to play in helping deliver more impactful learning, characterised by enhanced clarity, engagement

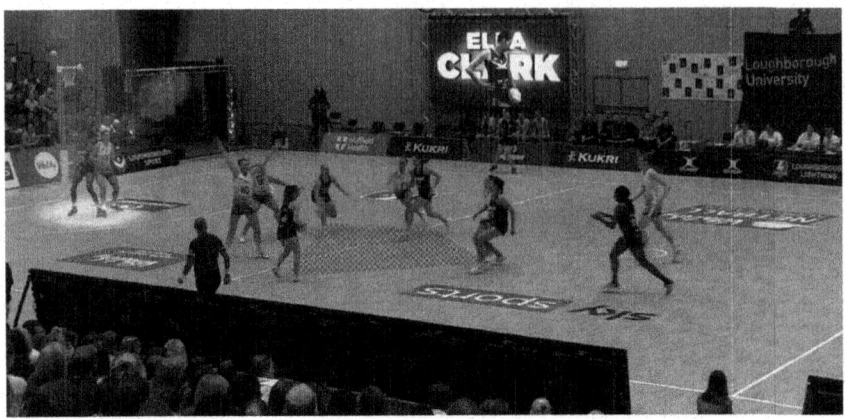

FIGURE 2.16   Telestrated video.

and retention of key information. Follow up empirical research by Smith et al. (2022) provides further positive evidence to the usefulness of telestration in aiding retention and enhancing learning. The telestration market has expanded considerably since the popularisation began, with many offers now available for analysts to select in their uptake and consideration of the tool in practice.

Hudl Studio

Those using Hudl SportsCode as their capture software can now quickly add in telestration to their video capture process. Their Studio (Figure 2.17) software allows users to quickly add professional and dynamic drawings to multiple angles within video packages. Studio sits as an external product to SportsCode, but integrates quickly to generate advanced and easy to use telestration.

Coach Paint

Claimed to be the most used product in elite football, coach paint supports teams in creating telestrated clips flexible for use in any workflow, on any operating system. The AI-enabled product allows automated player tracking in real time, whilst the automatic chroma keyer simplifies graphics workflows. Moveable 3D interacting tools enable the visualisation of bespoke images to help tell tactical stories in a fully configurable and editable timeline.

Metrica Play

An integrated coding and telestration software, Play by Metrica Sports claims to be a complete solution from coding through to player sharing. Available across multiple platforms, the software enables everything to be housed in a single place, coding, video editing and adding telestrations with a small number of

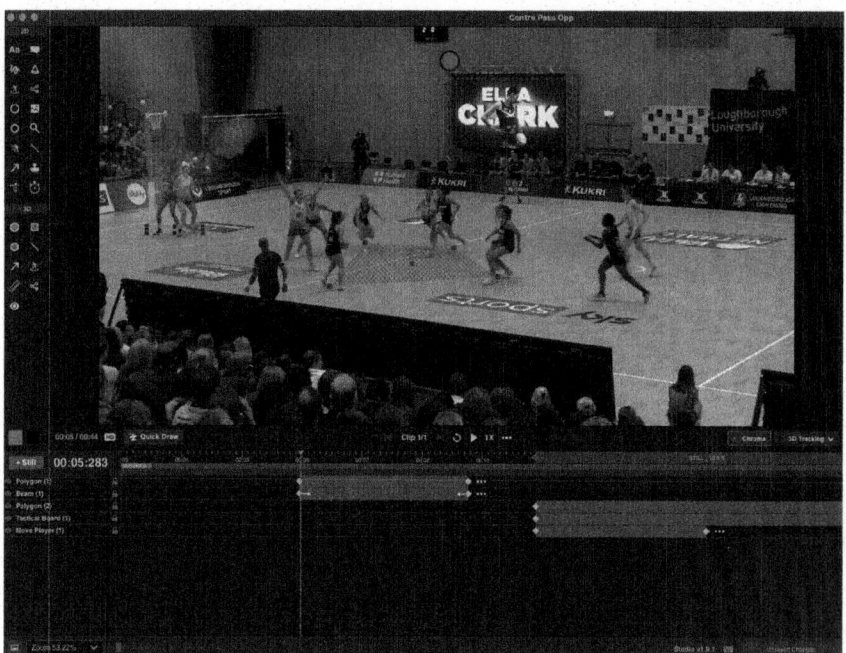

FIGURE 2.17 Hudl Studio.

clicks. Depending on the product purchased, Play offers an affordable solution which also enables some automated coding and tracking, version dependent. Heat mapping, live formation and online storage provide an integrated solution for multiple sports.

KlipDraw

A product of NacSport, KlipDraw seeks to provide eye-catching clear-cut illustrations on still frames and moving clips. At an affordable price, the analysis software is intuitive allowing for object and player tracking, animated graphics and customisable features. Working on Windows operating systems and integrating well with NacSport coding software, the product is well suited to lower-budget teams and individuals who still need a powerful visualisation tool.

Hosting Platforms

The advancement and increased use of internet technology has changed the way performance analysts deliver their feedback, opening up new global and remote feedback opportunities. Now available at times and locations to suit, mobile devices with apps are used extensively to report performance analysis feedback. These technologies are especially useful for travelling teams, where team bus or

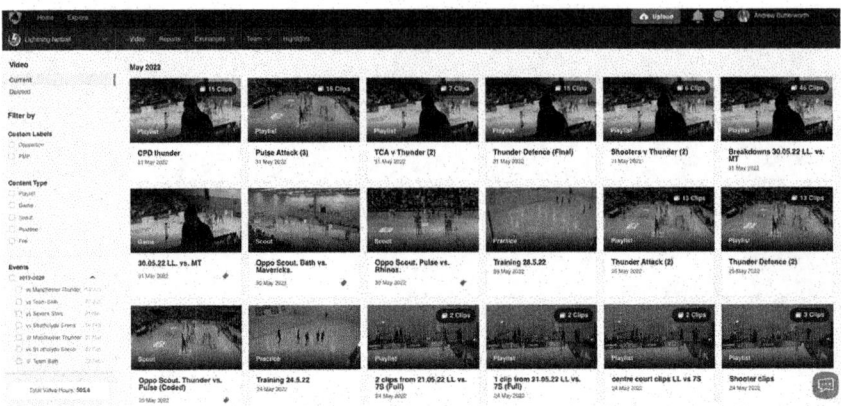

FIGURE 2.18 Hudl.com.

plane journeys can now be used in part for analysis, rather than the latest streaming series. The result of these technologies has meant increased engagement with performance analysis than would have been possible before this type of system was used (O'Donoghue & Mayes, 2013).

Hudl.com

Providing a single platform to host video and data concurrently, Hudl.com (Figure 2.18) allows users to upload their footage directly from Hudl SportsCode onto a dedicated platform that can be accessed anywhere, on any device. Permissions-based sharing means that those who should see the analysis do, with different permissions available for coaches and athletes to allow for specific analysis to be performed. Quickly sharing with these targeted groups allows for playlists to be sent with interactive video commenting and notes as another means for engagement. Hudl.com also offers reporting windows and shared video sessions whereby users on different devices can collaborate live to conduct analysis sessions. Offering easy to use apps for Android and Apple mobile devices, it can also be accessed via web browsers too. New integration back to Hudl SportsCode to simplify workflow processes are also now available, speeding up the integration of analysis completed online and on Mac.

Catapult Pro Video – Hub

Hub connects teams and provides an easy way to share video, reports and insights into performance in an online environment. After video and data are uploaded, Hub offers a powerful search and retrieval function which allows the tagged data to be easily accessed. Distribution of the clips can also be done easily within the web-based platform to ensure that the right people access content. Integrated with Focus, the Hub can also be used for sharing content live with the bench and sending additional materials. Additional post-match reports and documents can also be uploaded for easy sharing and syncing with those who need access.

Coach Logic

Introducing and involving players with the analysis process is central to the Coach Logic tool, which seeks to engage players with analysis and allow them to discover and learn. Using a feed feature, much like many social media outlets, content is posted for players to engage with using playlists of video, documents, messages and links, sent directly to groups or individuals. Further analysis features which allow for online tagging of core events is present which can then be sent to playlists and shared. Central to the Coach Logic platform is the desire to attempt further engagement by players in the analysis process by asking them to respond, comment and clip.

Sharimg

Sharimg is the hosting platform for video and data exported from NacSport, offering an online experience for users to upload video, data and documents. With permissions set by the administrator, the platform allows for collaboration and communication about key clips, whilst also allowing for presentations and matrixes to be created.

In-Play Online

In-Play is a video-based tool which offers some limited coding capabilities too. The system relies on users uploading their own footage, captured however they have chosen to do using any device that they have access to, and then storing on the cloud system. Analysts can then use a limited tagging suite to break down the captured video themselves on the online system. Alternatively, users can also import .xml files exported out from other capture software to sync online. When the process is completed, the platform offers video playlists to help with meetings and match de-briefs and compatibility access across multiple devices.

Data Sources

The advent of a more data-driven approach to performance analysis has seen huge changes in the way analysis is approached. The emergence of huge data has driven analytical practice, seeking to manipulate and create insights from a near infinite quantity of data points. There are now many different companies selling pre-coded data to teams and organisations seeking to intake volumes of data, seeking in return to harness the power of analytical insight. Opta, StatsBomb, Instat, FB Ref, Champion Data and STATS all offer significant volumes of data in a variety of sports. WyScout meanwhile is the world's largest football database with over 460,000 individual player profiles and 200,000 games from over 100 countries. Products such as this enable decision making to be faster, insights to be more elaborate and tactics to become more refined. The reliability, selection and procurement of any of these products remains open to end-user's interpretation, but there is no doubting the power that they harness.

Impact and Value

This chapter has outlined a number of the current technologies available to performance analysts, showcasing some of their particular features and potential implications into practice. The growth of new technologies being adopted by performance analysis shows no signs of slowing, with ever increasing capabilities, power and functions. Technology has undoubtedly changed performance analysis for the better, and challenged analysts to work in new and innovative manners for the betterment of performance. Research confirms this, with Brooks (2014) discovering that technologically driven environments result in better end-user outcomes than traditional settings. No doubt soon there will be further upgrades, more innovation, more automation, all in less time than now. But not all technologies are suitable or needed in the performance analysis sphere, and so whatever the face of technology looks like over the years to come, considerable thought must be given to the impact of it in the learning environment and on the end user.

Multifaceted, the learning environment comprises the diverse cultural, contextual and physical influences that may impact upon end user experience and learning. Culture is rich in every organisation and provides a welcome dynamic ecosystem of attitudes and values. These cultures bring about different views and uptakes of technology and impact the way that they can be implemented. Contextual factors meanwhile are the often-invisible collection of inter-connecting factors that impact on the successful completion of a role such as legal, micro-political, age dynamics, recent results, age and stage, with clear influences on the uptake and integration of technology. Meanwhile, the physical space and technologies that we use in our analysis feedback have a direct impact on behaviours, with Romina (2014) suggesting that the physical space impacts upon behaviour, motivation and learning outcomes. However, new technologies are very rarely planned around a specific pedagogical approach and instead there is an assumption that they will seamlessly integrate.

And so, do you *really* need a drone? Have the analysis team truly thought through the cost-benefit analysis of this tool for the impact upon athlete learning and the learning environment being created? Or is it procured because it can be, because your nearest rivals have one and because it looks good on the analyst's social media feeds? After all, given the current battery life, you can't even capture half of a game, and does anyone actually have a licence to fly it? Drones are just one example here and this is in no way saying that they are not a useful tool in the correct context. It is though to say that the use of any technology must be aligned with learning needs, pedagogy and feedback processes. Typically, the introduction of new IT technology is not planned around a pedagogical approach, which presents potential problems under these assumptions. Organisations with a raft of new technology but little planning behind the use of it will not make best use of it for the benefit of end users.

Comprehensive strategies therefore need to be designed to ensure the correct management and roll out of technology in line with core pedagogical principles and underlying learning concepts. The culture, context and physical environments must be considered in assessing their suitability for implementation into practice. If we fail to do this, there is a danger that the technology will outgrow us and that our feedback processes become clouded with confusion, complication and obstacles to learning. Nicholls et al. (2019) have already pointed to this, with their paper calling for a multi-disciplinary approach to advance our understanding of technological impact, with Ratten (2020) also discussing the need for strategy and management of technology. That though takes time, something which is all too precious in the cut and thrust of elite sport, with Barker-Ruchti et al. (2021) pointing to needing extra staff to help operate these technologies, though that does seem somewhat counterintuitive and contradictory to some of the automation features of the technologies we have examined in this chapter. If we are truly to move forwards in a collaborative and involved manner, armed with technology, we must do so with careful thought and clear rhyme behind our reason.

Concluding Remarks

The abundant rise of technology has no doubt aided in the efficiency of performance analysis, offering new opportunities and helping better inform coaches and players in valid and reliable manners. There are an exciting number of companies in the performance analysis technology market, all vying for club's money with the promise of enhanced performance possibilities. Each must be considered carefully in turn, aligning with club and coaching philosophies, understanding underpinning values to deliberate their value in individual contexts. Whichever are elected for use, they must remain cognisant of their place in the coaching process, not to replace, but to enhance, check and sometimes challenge. And so, despite the abundance of technologies, the most important remaining factor is the need to interpret the final output and translate the message back in tandem with key stakeholders in pedagogically appropriate manners.

References

Barker-Ruchti, N., Svensson, R., Svensson, D., & Fransson, D. (2021). Don't buy a pig in a poke: Considering challenges of and problems with performance analysis technologies in Swedish men's elite football. *Performance Enhancement & Health, 9*(1), 100191.

Bedir, D., & Erhan, S.E. (2021). The effect of virtual reality technology on the imagery skills and performance of target-based sports athletes. *Frontiers in Psychology, 11*, 2073.

Bideau, B., Kulpa, R., Vignais, N., Brault, S., & Multon, F. (2010). Using virtual reality to analyse sport performance. *IEEE Computer Graphics and Applications, 30*(2), 14–21.

Brooks, C. (2014). Space matters: the impact of formal learning environments on student learning. *British Journal of Educational Technology, 42*(5), 719–726.

Butterworth, A.D., Turner, D.J., & Johnstone, J. (2012). Coaches perceptions of the potential use of performance analysis in badminton. *International Journal of Performance Analysis in Sport, 12*(2), 452–467.

Cabrillo, S., & Dahms, S. (2018). How strategic management drives intellectual capital to superior innovation and market performance. *Journal of Knowledge Management, 22*(3), 621–648.

Ericsson, C. & Horgby, C.E.B. (2020). Women and commercial football in Sweden. In *Women and commercial football in Sweden*. Retrieved 2nd July 2022, from: https://idrottsforum.org/ericsson-horgby200921-in-english/

Franks, I.M., & Miller, G. (1986). Eyewitness testimony in sport. *Journal of Sport Behaviour, 9*, 39–45.

Hutchins, B., & Rowe, D. (2013). *Digital media sport: Technology, power and culture in the network society*. Oxon: Routledge.

Jones, D., Rands, S., & Butterworth, A.D. (2020). The use and perceived value of telestration tools in elite football. *International Journal of Performance Analysis in Sport, 20*(3), 373–388.

Laird, P., & Waters, L. (2008). Eye witness recollection of sports coaches. *International Journal of Performance Analysis in Sport, 8*(1), 76–84.

Mallen, C. (2019). *Emerging technologies in sport: Implications for sport management*. Oxon: Routledge.

Mitchell, J., Maratos, F.A., Giles, D., Taylor, N., Butterworth, A.D., & Sheffield, D. (2020). The visual search strategies underpinning effective observational analysis in the coaching of climbing movement. *Frontiers in Psychology, 11*, 1025.

Nicholls, S.B., James, N., Bryant, E. & Wells, J. (2019). The implementation of performance analysis and feedback within Olympic sport: The performance analyst's perspective. *International Journal of Sports Science & Coaching, 14*(1), 63–71.

O'Donoghue, P., & Mayes, A. (2013). Performance analysis, feedback and communication. In T. McGarry, P. O'Donoghue & J. Sampaio (Eds.), *Routledge handbook of sports performance analysis* (pp. 155–164). London: Routledge.

Ratten, V. (2020). Sport technology: A commentary. *The Journal of High Technology Management Research, 31*(1), 100383.

Riot, C., & James, D. (2013). Innovating to grow: The wider context of innovation in sport. *Proceedings of ASTN, 1*(1), 40–42.

Romina, A. (2014). Students perceptions of the condition of their classroom and physical learning environment. *College Student Journal, 48*(4), 714–723.

Smith, J., Rands, S., Bateman, M., & Francis, J. (2022). Assessing the efficacy of video telestration in aiding memory recall among elite professional football players. *Sports Innovation Journal, 3*, 61–81.

Trabal, P. (2013). Resistence to technological innovation in elite sport. *International Review for the Sociology of Sport, 43*(3), 313–330.

Zeimers, G., Anagnostopoulos, C., Zintz, T., & Willem, A. (2019). Organisational learning for social corporate responsibility in sport organisations. *European Sport Management Quarterly, 19*(1), 80–101.

3

PERFORMANCE ANALYSIS IN AN INTERDISCIPLINARY SPORT SCIENCE TEAM

Andrew Butterworth

Introduction

Many interchangeable terms and acronyms are used as the collective noun for a group of sports science practitioners working across multiple disciplines. Sport science team (SST) is one such term, sport science and sport medicine (SSSM) team another. In addition, multi- and inter-disciplinary teams are now heard as common place too, often also referred to solely by their acronyms of MDT or IDT. Whilst these are commonly referred to as an aspiration for working practice, they are not always fully understood and that aspiration all too often never comes to fruition. Instead practitioners often remain working in their silos, in a form of mono-disciplinary practice. Performance analysts are often tasked with working towards either MDT or IDT practice too and whilst aspirational, it is difficult to do so unless they know the accurate definition of these and understand *how* and importantly *why*, they are trying to work in that manner.

The importance of this content cannot be understated, with one of these working practices now common place in a majority of environments. There are, for example, many job adverts now which will ask candidates to be aware of or able to evidence understanding or working within MDT or IDT environments. Given the ever-increasing popularity of our profession and competition for roles, it is perhaps the deeper knowledge and understanding of these such areas, beyond the technical knowledge and understanding, that might help be the differential. And so, if we are to gain that job role, we must have a clear appreciation of what these working practices are and how to work within them.

Therefore, this chapter will first define and provide practical examples of each of these working practices in turn using an applied fictional example, before going on to discuss the value of each in situ in an elite sporting environment. Performance analysis will be carefully considered for each, discussing the ways

DOI: 10.4324/9781003226659-3

in which practitioners might be able to collaborate with other sport science disciplines. With IDT working seen as the gold standard, critically this chapter will then consider how to work towards this structure of support, specifically considering the performance analysts role in collaborating with other sport science disciplines, and the intended outcomes.

Defining Working Practices

Working in sport will provide a number of challenges and situations which require the support of one or more sports science practitioners. Our ultimate role of course is to help our end users (e.g. coaches and athletes) towards a better performance outcome, and so in attempting to achieve that outcome, we must attempt to solve any challenges that come our way. When a problem or task occurs, it will require the support of the sports science team to solve it. Given that research (e.g. Gould & Damarjian, 1998) demonstrates that optimal performance is founded upon technical, tactical, physical and mental performance combined, it is unlikely that single individuals will have the requisite knowledge to cover all of these areas.

Therefore, the organisational structure that is in place will likely consist of a number of practitioners in different disciplines. For some, usually at the very elite end of sport, this will consist of many disciplines such as strength and conditioning, psychology, biomechanics, physiology, nutrition and performance analysis. For others though, money is an issue which restricts from having such a high number of specialists, and so support is somewhat more limited. Regardless of how many practitioners and roles there are though, how (or indeed if) these disciplines come together to see how that problem can be solved, will vary from team to team.

There are three frequently cited ways of working which can be used to help find a solution to the common problem; mono-, multi- and inter-disciplinary practice, each typified by a number of different characteristics. The latter two are often used interchangeably and frequently aspired towards by teams, though often this is without really understanding the definition of each or the important differences between them. For newly forming or re-developing SSTs, knowledge of the remits of each of these working manners is important, equally as it is for those aspiring to work in such manners. Though it is not as simple as electing a working model and then operating in that way, and there are a number of considerations and challenges that will need to be contemplated. There are both internal and external factors that influence the manner of working, not least including socio-economic factors but also contextual and cultural impacts too.

In helping define, explain and work through the practice of each of these approaches, we'll use the same fictional mock problem as outlined below. The problem will be 'solved' under the guise of each approach in turn, showcasing examples of practice that might be utilised. We'll also consider the differences between each approach and what changes between each, a form of gap analysis.

The (Fictional) Problem

A creative midfield football player has returned from a serious knee injury, having progressed well through initial rehabilitation. However, on their return, the player is struggling for form and has had a number of under par performances. The player has also struggled to complete 90 minutes and has been substituted around 60 minutes into each match. Outside of football, the player has just moved house and had a young child. The sport science staff at the football club have been tasked with uncovering what is causing the poor form, in an attempt to return the player to a higher level of performance.

Defining Mono-Disciplinary Practice

Mono-disciplinary practice is characterised by single sport science disciplines working in silo. Support for athletes in this manner is provided by a single sports science discipline on its own, attempting to solve the problem using their discipline knowledge only. In practice this means using either the psychology *or* physiology *or* performance analysis practitioners (or indeed any other of the sport sciences) on their own, tasking them with finding a solution to the problem. In this manner of working most often the discipline to be used is dictated by those higher in the organisation, or a practitioner decides to take full ownership, believing that their discipline is the one which can be most useful to solving the issue at hand. This provides a very narrow field of vision and constricts the available information when making decisions about how to solve a problem. It is unlikely that a single person or single discipline holds a sufficient depth of knowledge to create an optimal performance solution.

Solving Our Problem with Mono-Disciplinary Practice

Our fictional problem is multi-faceted, with a number of potential explanations of why the player has not returned to full form since returning. If we were to work as performance analysts in a mono-disciplinary manner to solve it, we would utilise only our own knowledge and expertise and tools available to us. No other disciplines would be involved in investigating this problem and it would be fully assigned to ourselves.

Working in this manner, given that the problem outlines poor form, it would be first beneficial to undertake a comparison piece to establish the performance indicator values pre- and post-injury. The performance analyst could compare data sets from before and after in an attempt to identify areas of concern. If data is available, it would be beneficial to do this over multiple matches using performance profiling techniques. This would help understand any other outside contextual inferences and also provide a more informed and objective overview of pre- and post-injury. The use of profiling would also help uncover any consistencies or inconsistencies in specific variables that might also help explain the poor form.

Whilst this approach would provide us with information on *what* is happening with the players performance indicator data, it gives us very limited information regarding *why* the values have dropped. It is helpful that the analyst is able to uncover what areas are concerning and which need attention, but they are not able to provide a deep insight into *why*. This is where the mono-disciplinary approach is very limited in its usefulness for real-world practice, as the knowledge base being used is constricted solely to performance analysis data. To solve this problem and uncover some of the reasons why the performance indicator values have dropped, other sport science disciplines are required.

Defining Multi-disciplinary Practice

Multi-disciplinary practice (MDT) working involves multiple people and multiple disciplines of sports science each working on solutions to a common problem in parallel. Using this model of working, two or more disciplines would each attempt to uncover more information on a common problem, and find solutions using their discipline. This means that we would have a physiologist and a performance analyst working on the same problem (and any other relevant disciplines too). By its very nature, MDT working involves multiple disciplines and so there is a need for some level of communication and information sharing between the disciplines. This communication usually comes in the form of information sharing after each discipline has undertaken their own work first. At this point, they can compare each of their findings and proposed interventions to devise a way forward to resolve the problem.

Solving Our Problem with MDT Practice

Given that our problem is multi-faceted and the mono-disciplinary work of the performance analyst does not give us the full picture, our MDT practice draws upon knowledge of other disciplines too, in an attempt to try and help uncover some of the *why* behind what is found. In the MDT, the role of the performance analyst would stay largely the same as in the mono-disciplinary approach, by undertaking informed comparisons to uncover where areas of attention lie. The difference in the MDT approach is that once they have been communicated, based upon the findings of the other sport sciences, will be in communication with the other discipline(s) about their findings. These might correlate with the other disciplines or be conflicting and so conversations will have to ensue. The analyst might then be asked to complete additional work to help inform the decision making process. Equally, the analyst might also want to ask for additional information from other disciplines before sharing that back.

In addition to our performance analysis work, our mock problem includes noticeable elements in the players game related to psychology, physiology, strength and conditioning and nutrition. Since the player is struggling to complete more than 60 minutes of a game, it is highly likely that the physiologist will look to conduct further investigations and testing as to the players capacity to perform, the strength and conditioning coach might also consider the appropriateness of the gym programme and assessing the GPS data to try and identify any issues and increase capacity. Given that there are also personal situations in our case study example, the psychologist might be interested in speaking with the player too and considering if any strategies might be employed to enhance the mindset of the player or working with a performance lifestyle or liaison officer. Under the MDT approach, each discipline does their work in their silo's working independently of each other, before bringing together the findings later on. They would communicate and discuss once the individual mono-disciplinary interventions have been made first.

The addition of other sports science disciplines in helping our player will yield more information and potentially help us uncover the *why* behind the poor form. In returning that information to the performance analysts, there might then be interesting information that needs further investigation or intervention. For example, if the strength and conditioning coach assesses the GPS data, they might reveal that the player is not making as many high-speed runs as they were pre-injury, that their recovery runs are not walking and not jogging, and that the total distance covered is also significantly less. This additional information is now of interest to other disciplines, not least the physiologist for their capacity investigations, so too the nutritionist to assess if fuelling strategies are appropriate.

For performance analysis, the additional information garnered then offers up the opportunity to help provide answers to the *why* questions posed by others, by providing further evidence to help understand. The analysts will be able to provide video footage that shows where on the pitch and when in the game the high-speed runs were being made previously, and comparing that to video of more recent games, highlighting where opportunities to do so are not being taken up. They can also provide situational and contextually informed opposition tactical insights which might be restricting the player from performing the same actions, or show opportunities that are not being taken. This information will prove valuable to the other sport sciences, in helping them understand what underpins the numbers they have from their tests and so start to consider more

Equally, the data from the other sport sciences might help answer the analysts own *why*, helping to contextualise and understand the reasons behind some of the lower performance indicator values. Reasons might owe to physiological capacity not being as high, or poor nutrition strategies or a shift in psychology which has impacted on pitch performance. By the other disciplines returning this information to us, this will likely result in an additional piece of work for the analysts to do, seeking to identify these reasons why, and then deliver further suggestions for interventions. The advent of an MDT approach where data come together after initial mono-disciplinary work, helps us to understand the underpinning reasons behind performance levels and the reasons for the poor form. It is this approach which helps us towards a fuller holistic understanding of our problem, though there is still more collaboration and mutual work that can be done to enhance interventions and get our player back to form.

Defining Inter-disciplinary Practice

Inter-disciplinary practice (IDT) working is the involvement of multiple people and disciplines working collaboratively together on a common problem from the outset. The term *IDT* describes a group of professionals from many different disciplines cooperating in tandem to work on a common goal with the same athlete. It is this practice which will see multiple disciplines interacting fully in order to help solve the problem. The distinction between MDT and IDT is that before any testing or interventions are undertaken by the individual disciplines, full collaboration and agreement are sought. Rather than in an MDT approach where each discipline will work in silo until their work is complete and information sharing begins, IDT working starts with collaborative conversations and specifically targets disciplines to collaborate together in undertaking their information gathering. It is this conversation which places IDT apart, and it is that practice which helps us to answer our *why* questions in a holistic manner, encompassing all required disciplines.

IDT working requires a very strong working relationship, in order that information may be shared and integrated together from multiple sources, for the benefit of the end user. Cross comparisons with data sets from multiple disciplines in various mediums will be made, alongside the full integration and universal sharing of the information made available. This integration provides a better outcome for the athlete since each discipline is considered in collaboration and built in as part of the overall response and interventions prescribed. With IDT working, SSTs will use this strong working relationship and collaborate from the outset, meaning that all available sciences will have the opportunity to suggest and put forward solutions from their discipline in turn. Each will be carefully considered and information synthesis and critically challenged in order to reach the optimal outcome, with an intervention strategy decided upon. Communication is vital to this, ensuring that open and honest conversations can be facilitated to air all of the important information. There is also a need for mutual trust and understanding alongside confidentiality, given that potentially sensitive personal information about an athlete might be shared.

Solving Our Problem with IDT Practice

We have already established that our problem requires the intervention of multiple sports science disciplines. Under the MDT approach, we suggested that there is a need for different sciences to investigate given the multifaceted and complex nature of the problem at hand, though the amalgamation of that information is only done towards the end of the process. In solving our problem with an IDT, members will first seek to fully understand the problem at hand, asking each discipline in turn to provide their initial assessment. Given that this is now being done in a holistic manner, one of our first steps might be looking back to the initial injury and the rehabilitation programme prescribed to ascertain if any lessons can be learnt from that, or if anything there is impacting performance now.

The initial role of the performance analyst here may be to provide video footage of the injury again from multiple angles, syncing and ordering this appropriately to stimulate conversation. The analyst might also ascertain any factors that led to the injury (e.g. phase of play, position on pitch, opposition involvement) and extract performance indicator data on the level at which the athlete was performing pre injury. Using this information in conversation, the physiotherapy and strength and conditioning experts will discuss in collaboration with other members, ensuring that all aspects of the players injury have been considered, also considering with the psychologist any leading factors.

Having done so, focus might shift to ascertaining if that initial rehabilitation programme and physical markers produced has had any impact upon the players form now. The physiologist would also be part of these conversations, understanding how the capacity of the athlete has been rebuilt during that rehabilitation phase, and suggesting what might be needed now. For the performance analyst, the role here might be to provide video and numerical data of technical skills associated with the player, captured prior to injury and since the initial rehabilitation process. In doing so this might use performance profiling methods to uncover specific areas of the players game which are performing worse than pre-injury. This forms a valuable opportunity to ascertain what the problem is, before others in the IDT can then help with understanding *why* that is.

Answering the *why* involves the numerous disciplines again, with each having the opportunity to input their observations based upon the data identified by the analyst. Collaborative conversations in meetings and informally will ensure that practitioners each input their suggested interventions for getting the player back into form. Before any actions or interventions are decided upon, all information will have been considered in turn and decisions made by coaches as to the most appropriate strategy. Our applied example might find that the player is making fewer forward runs, undertaking less high intensity movements and failing to play as many through balls as pre-injury. Mini sub-teams may form and disciplines are asked to work closely with each other on certain aspects of that intervention. The analysts and psychologists might form one of these, working towards goal setting, imagery and motivational interventions for the athlete to increase confidence to play those through balls, whilst strength and conditioning, nutrition and physiotherapy collaborate to design physical training blocks to increase capacity for high intensity movements and forward runs. Information from each sub team is then driven back into the wider IDT for final discussion and decision on timelines, communication and playing minutes.

A further role for the analyst within this IDT solution might be to undertake a gap analysis and detail data and information on others who can play in the same position. Given that our player is out of form, as part of the IDT's decision making, they might feel it is better to rest the player whilst additional training and rehabilitation are undertaken. And so, if others have to fill that position, the analyst can help provide knowledge and insight about who might be best placed to come into the side, based upon profiling insight and opposition knowledge, also linked to the specific contextual needs ahead of upcoming matches. This process will also involve others within the IDT who will discuss the decision based on their own holistic understanding of the athletes who could replace. This practice all revolves centrally around collaboration, communication and information sharing, in an attempt to utilise aspirational best practice workflows.

Seen as the gold standard of sport science practice, IDT working requires a number of critical success factors. Interaction, information sharing and trust are all vital. By its very nature, IDT practice involves numerous disciplines, not just performance analysts and so the direction of this chapter now seeks to provide practical recommendations for *why* and *how* we encourage moving towards that manner of working. In doing so, a number of disciplines will be considered, and how to work with them especially since as analysts we must learn more about them. And so, the section serves as a guide for enhancing performance analyst's knowledge of how to work in the IDT, with a core focus on the specifics that performance analysts can consider, whilst also touching upon the other sciences and collaboration opportunities.

Towards IDT Practice

Why

If a sustained and meaningful effort is made to enhance working practice towards IDT characteristics, then there is a growing body of evidence which highlights the value and worth of doing so. Holistically, the value of IDT practice allows practitioners to collaborate and so better understand individualised and team athletic performances in a more inclusive manner. Empirical research into the area is also helping practitioners to understand the importance of dedicating time to setting up IDT working intricacies and practices to lead towards successful outcomes.

That success is multifaceted and might come in a variety of forms, for example improved indicator values, on-pitch achievements, enhanced talent ID, better informed player development pathways, and increased practice and knowledge for the practitioner. Each of these successes relies on more information being made available, to allow sharing and better insights to be drawn, something which is advocated in the early literature by Burwitz et al. (1994) who suggest that an IDT approach provides information that would not be normally available under other manners of working. For example, if mono–disciplinary working is utilised (where information sharing does not take place), the information and conversation that are generated when the disciplines cross compare their data would not happen and such information would remain constricted. Given that sport performance is so dynamic with many interacting elements combining to produce performance, if information from any of those elements is missing or not generated at all, then the potential for enhanced performance is limited as the constraints interact with each other.

If disciplines were working in silo, one might suggest one intervention which conflicts with that of another, resulting in confusion for the athlete. For example, a player might be struggling with confidence, and so in silo the performance analyst decides to produce a motivational video of the players best bits set to music. Separately, the psychologist is holding conversations with the player but decides that the best intervention would be to encourage self-talk and physical relaxation given that over arousal is a potential issue. These two decisions conflict, with the analyst's intervention likely to over arouse the athlete further, but the psychologists seeking to reduce that. The result could then be confusion for the athlete and further poor performances. IDT working removes this possibility for contradictory advice, ensuring that from the outset, information is shared in an interactive manner across all disciplines. It is this interaction that comes with an IDT approach which ensures there is no conflict in the interventions proposed and that resultantly appropriate steps are suggested.

Talent ID is also said to be improved by an IDT approach to sport science, given that information sharing is prevalent and conversations help to lessen contrasting advice and conflict (Burwitz et al., 1994). The role of performance analysis in Talent ID is well documented in practice and empirical literature, especially given the objective data that the analysts can help provide. Combining the valuable data analysts produce on individual athletes, benchmarking and undertaking trend analyses using performance profiling methods is an interesting way of keeping track of developing progress. Utilising that data further in an IDT manner with other disciplines will further enhance this practice for developing and aspiring athletes. As profiles are created and other disciplines begin their work too, the IDT approach would see physical and psychological data amongst others combined into conversations about development plans and pathway design. Buekers et al. (2016) suggest similar, advising that such an integrated approach provides a better profile of each athlete that results in targeted interventions to improve successful outcomes.

The dynamic nature of sport is multifaceted, with many interactive and moving parts resulting in end outcomes for athletes. The environment in which the sport is performed and other contextual variables such as opposition, venue, score line and match importance all impact the performance. Given this complexity and these number of outside influences, a further benefit that IDT practice brings is the collaboration of knowledge and a better understanding of these environmental factors. Understanding them more using multiple disciplines in an IDT working model allows practitioners and coaches to provide a more holistic intervention, cognisant of influencing dynamics. In Canadian sport for example, the prevalence of IDT working is well documented, with two key remits being to achieve podium performances and promote the holistic development of athletes (Piggott et al., 2018). Other research evidence promotes this too, with Lozano et al.'s (2020) educational-based paper suggesting that learning in an interdisciplinary manner, entwined with technological tools promotes greater motivation and better understanding of content.

Coaches too cite the benefits of IDT practice, with Williams and Kendall (2007) reporting that the coaches they interviewed believe IDT practice better informs training programmes. It is this information sharing and informed practice which provide real value to be added to coaches and athletes' performances alike. Earlier research by Willimczik (1992) also accentuated the importance of collaborative IDT working in helping impact coaching science by accepting the need to embrace each discipline to produce an overarching strategy. And so, given these many benefits and values that IDT working provides to sport science practitioners, to coaches and to athletes, it is perhaps not surprising that there is a shift towards this working manner. Piggott et al. (2018) for example cite that more and more sports science teams are attempting to make this move, discovering that an increasing percentage of practice is IDT. The growing knowledge base of evidence for the worth of the practice, alongside better working collaborations, is aiding this move for practitioners and athletes alike.

Barriers and Reluctance

Though seen as an aspirational working practice, and the prevalence is growing (e.g. Piggott et al., 2018), some empirical reviews of the sport science literature have suggested that IDT practice is not as widespread as expected, or hoped in some quarters. Buekers et al. (2016) suggest that IDT research practice is scarce, summarising that more is required. Contemplating the reasons why this might be, Piggott et al. (2018) suggest that frameworks, organisational preference and resources might be negatively contributing factors. Awareness is critical, with many practitioners in the field having heard or used the buzz words or acronyms of MDT or IDT, but not fully understanding what they are or how to work towards them. Frameworks to underpin and guide IDT working practice have been scarce and so the field has not been able to progress as quickly as hoped. IDT working is dependent upon individual practitioners being highly organised, collaborating and cooperating with each other, requiring high levels of inter dependence, trust and information sharing. If that sharing is not free flowing and abundant, issues will likely occur, given that the full picture cannot be ascertained with data missing. If any one member of the SST is more withdrawn and prefers a mono-disciplinary approach, the success of the final holistic intervention reduces. The resources required to undertake IDT practice outweigh those of a mono approach, with a number of important considerations required. The physical meeting and sharing and sharing of information are resources in themselves, and so too are the actual mechanisms by which information will be stored and shared, all whilst maintaining version control and data currency.

To be successful, an IDT approach requires personal commitment by each practitioner. Given that working in an IDT manner takes time, concerted effort and ongoing learning, perhaps it is not wholly surprising that it is yet to be fully embedded. After all, the mono role in itself is usually demanding enough, and so finding the effort and motivation to engage in learning outside of analysis, unless it is built explicitly into the job description, can be difficult. Given that IDT practice requires collaboration, meeting and sharing, it also comes with a need to provide some training or insight to others about what the role actually entails and what is produced, all of which take time too. As we are only too acutely aware, technology is embedded in our roles, teaching others this is time consuming, as is learning other technologies that other practitioners use too. Whilst time is the most obvious barrier, others may have an unwillingness or reluctance to change from current practice. Opening up our analysis world to outsiders from other sport science disciplines might be an alien concept to some. Performance analysis is usually shrouded in secrecy, even within an organisation and so fears of intrusion and a loss of control over process may occur. This might also lead to a fear of role clarity being lost and blurred lines as to who is responsible for what. And in talking of responsibility, another consideration is who leads, drives and implements the IDT approach and who is ultimately responsible for bringing together the IDT collaborations.

And so, if practitioners are to work in an IDT manner, they must overcome these barriers, re-consider their reluctances and seek solutions to ensure that the important data sharing and collaborative properties of IDT practice can be attained. Willingness and successfully navigating the interacting constraints of IDT practice is key to ensuring success. Clear organisational structures must be in place to allow for the ethical and morally fair sharing of data, whilst roles and responsibilities for each practitioner in the IDT should be outlined from the beginning. If attained then this practice should help bring about some of the many cited benefits and values of IDT practice.

How

Performance analysis has previously been described by O'Donoghue and Mayes (2013) as a form of superglue between disciplines, enabling and helping to bring together the other sciences in attempting to work in an interdisciplinary manner. Given the information sharing properties of the discipline and the ability to deliver informed insights into practice from both data and video sources, it is perhaps not surprising that analysts are sometimes also referred to as *The Informer*. This information sharing and collaboration back in as part of the IDT is vital, and so knowing how to work as an inter-disciplinary performance analysis practitioner is growing importance for the analyst's professional toolkit. This chapter has already provided information and understanding of what and why IDT practice is importance, and so there is then a need to understand *how* an analyst can seek to develop towards that gold standard practice.

Whilst some skills and knowledge are transferrable across disciplines, much of the specialist information and understanding of individual sciences is specialist and bespoke to each. Equally, given the vast amounts of empirical research emerging in each science, the knowledge and practice of each is continually evolving too, and in turn transforming practical implementation. And so, asking numerous disciplines of sport science to work in harmony with each other might seem like somewhat of a difficult task. However, the importance of this process should not be understated for the betterment of end-user performance. Collaborating and being willing to open up, share and co-operate with each discipline is positive though, and significantly, helps to build a common root of knowledge. It is this newly generated specialist information that can then be included in the interventions and recommendations put forwards for implementation with the athlete. In attempting to move to IDT working, there are important developments for performance analysts to consider, which as below will be explained.

Restructuring Practice

The technology and practices in the discipline of performance analysis are ever evolving, characterised in Chapter 2 of this book, which highlighted the growing number of technologies in our discipline. It also highlighted the importance of knowing *why* a certain technology is being embedded and critically, forming it around a pedagogical approach. The same is true of our working practice as analysts, whereby we must ensure that we are consistently updating our practice to reflect the ongoing needs. This requires a level of humbleness to change, and a willingness to put ourselves in a vulnerable position.

A key part of that change is firstly reflection, considering if our practice is suitable for the context in which we work, and if it is suitably open enough for collaboration and true IDT practice to take place. When we take a step back to examine our practice, we have the opportunity to be humble and honest, changing areas of habit or routine that we may have slipped into. The work we complete as performance analysts cannot be so factual and practical that we believe it is the only truth, and the only way to complete the task. Indeed, if we were to do so, the creativity and innovation that underpin it are lost, especially since sporting performance is so dynamic and a certain sense of mystery remains. There may be areas of our everyday coding and data extraction practice that are becoming outdated or inefficient, that we need to update in order to progress further. It might also be that those methods limit our interaction with psychology for example, since their use of quantiative data in its rawest form, is not as well versed.

In the spirit of IDT practice, Szabo and Tolnay (2016) discuss that restructuring our approaches, to help find solutions to our problems, might be achieved by borrowing from one discipline and transposing to another. To do so, we might then need to consider how other disciplines report their findings and then re-build our output windows or report back our findings to other members of the IDT in a clearer manner, in order that they can better comprehend our insights which in turn might lead to better synthesis between disciplines. A dynamic exploration of practice, grounded in context, will help to uncover areas that can be enhanced and the lines between disciplines to be intentionally blurred. Developing these key syntheses between disciplines offers respectful opportunities to enable integration and collaborative practice. This takes humbleness, openness to change and unpretentious practitioners who want the best overall outcome, rather than the easy solution or any feelings of positional threat.

Engelberg (1995) discusses this, stating that integration requires learning from others and being ok with feeling vulnerable. This research goes on to suggest that with an air of honesty, there should be less feelings of vulnerability and fearing that limitations might be found, but more of a positive mindset in discovery of strength and collaboration for the greater good. Rather than fearing being found out, the opposite should be true, where practitioners are positively recognised for losing their sense of security and being willing to change, restructure their practice and get lost in the mystery (Balague et al., 2016).

Knowledge Building and Professional Curiosity

In being humble and open to change, there is also a requirement for individual performance analysis practitioners to learn and build knowledge outside of their own discipline. To be able to work in an IDT manner, different disciplines need to communicate and be integrated, often with methodologies that require mastery from all involved. For this to be successful, there is a certain level of knowledge required by each practitioner of their professional counterparts. That is not to say that as performance analysts you must retrain, undertake numerous qualifications and become an expert in all other sciences, but it is to say that a base knowledge is important. It is no coincidence that University courses offer the first year as a grounding knowledge year, building up multi-disciplinary knowledge so that there is a base understanding, before they specialise their knowledge in years two and three. That same process is true of performance analysis specific courses, where students will typically study coaching, psychology, anatomy, physiology and biomechanics in their first year, before then enhancing their performance analysis specific knowledge beyond that.

It is this kind of deliberate approach grounded in a professional curiosity to learning that helps the IDT build a well-rounded approach to the application and contribution of knowledge. Szabo and Tolnay (2016) detail that true integration is achieved through the application and combination of different disciplines knowledge, building bridges between the specialist practitioners and disciplines for the betterment of end user outcome. And as Buekers et al. (2019) further explain, complications and performance problems are vast and wide ranging, and whilst the technology is now available to use and analytical methods also well embedded in many settings, the biggest remaining challenge is if the practitioners themselves, you reading this book now, are willing to continue learning and embrace learning with others.

The importance of this cannot be underestimated, especially since now the majority of job descriptions will ask for evidence of applicants being able to work in an IDT environment. Frequently examples will be asked for to ensure that the practitioner can collaborate with others and will not be siloed on their own, indeed in the case of the performance analyst, this is to ensure that the applicant won't be akin to the cliché of working in a darkened room alone!

Frameworks and Management

Messy, complicated and socially derived are just three mannerisms that simultaneously describe the coaching process and attempting to work in an IDT manner. With IDT part of the coaching process, this is perhaps unsurprising, and even more unsurprising that when we try to integrate multiple people with multiple skill sets over different problems and try to solve them, that things don't always work out according to plan. But interestingly, perhaps it is that last word, *plan*, which is most vital here, especially since it is often stated that performance analysis practice too is messy and unstructured in nature, often being reactive rather than proactive.

Resultantly, there needs to be more structure and framing to IDT practice, alongside clear management and responsibility for the overall approach. Suggestions have been made (e.g. Lozano et al., 2020) that there is a need to develop such frameworks of professional practice for working in IDT collaborations, since these are skills that are highly demanded in the current practice of performance analysis and sports science more generally. In developing this, there is a need for the important element of managerial structure and responsibility to be considered, which can influence the process. For an IDT to be successful, there is a need for an individual to have overarching responsibility for its design and running. Whilst most typically this will be the head coach or manager, it is sometimes too delegated out to senior sports science team members, performance directors or heads of sport science. Each organisation will need to consider who this person is, especially since they will likely be the person who aids in the initial development of the working framework. This leader will enable and facilitate IDT practice, driving toward deeper insight. Further help might come in the form of technology, with some having been developed to streamline practice, Kitman Labs one of the first bespoke offers to help integrate multiple sets of data together across the IDT, though coming at a fairly significant price.

There is then a need for practitioners to consider two elements to this framing of practice; the working IDT model itself, and the professional practitioners undertaking the work. For each, a model is important to help guide and structure working practice, whilst simultaneously ensuring that individuals know their role and how their important work contributes to the overall picture. And so, a working model of the IDT should be developed to ensure that role clarity is apparent and there is clear structure to how each evolving problem will be approached, how and when information will be shared and who will make the final decisions. Such a framework will help guide practice and design of interventions, an incentive to produce a comprehensive understanding of the performance environments. This will consider the initial collaborative and overarching conversations involved, and the role of each discipline in developing integrative interventions. This framework should also include the important logistical elements of when, how and where the IDT will meet, alongside practical details and timing considerations. The conversations that ensue should also be framed, ensuring that practitioners are aware of the boundaries of conversation, when it is and isn't appropriate to challenge and maintaining the core elements of sports science delivery. It should be rigid enough to guide practice and provide structure, but flexible enough to harness creativity and respond to the dynamic and evolving nature of sport without suffocating innovation. The model should not and cannot be dictated solely by research or modelling from other environments, since each is so dynamic and individual, and so the approach must be bespoke, with collaboration at the centre.

Summarising Practical Advice for Practice

IDT working is established as a working practice that should be desired, especially given its many benefits cited in this chapter and beyond. Those working in elite settings now, or seeking to in the future should be especially cognisant of these important factors in enhancing their understanding and ability to work within an IDT. First, start with the *why,* e.g. the underpinning reasons that have dictated the problem that has surfaced and how that problem can be solved. Think about the *why* from your own performance analysis perspective, and then think about it from others, considering the other impacting factors that might have caused it. This is the start of collaboration and openness, vital to success of the IDT.

Secondly, be humble, ask questions and be strong enough to put yourself in a position of professional vulnerability. It is here, when we learn more about others and other disciplines that professional growth really kicks on, and further opportunities to collaborate and grow your own knowledge surface. Maintaining curiosity and a willingness to continually learn, using reflection as an aid is especially important, and so draw (and increase) upon your knowledge of other sport sciences and consider where the two can work together for a deeper understanding of performance, and getting our athlete back to form. Ask to work with others who you would not normally and promote and IDT approach yourself, no matter how small that might seem. Those small and subtle changes, integrated with other disciplines, can add up to bigger interventions in time, after all, that is what IDT practice is grounded upon.

Concluding Remarks

The abundant rise of IDT working practices has been showcased in empirical research and applied practice. It is hoped that for the performance analysis community, this chapter helps aid that knowledge, understanding and working practice. Solving our common problem together in collaboration is proven to have significant benefits in a number of ways. The mutual cooperation and willingness to learn to enhance sport science practice increase professional efficacy and improve end user outcomes. For performance analysts, IDT practice is important as it can help us to better understand *why* something is happening and the reasons that underpin the performance indicator values that are being exhibited. It is with this sharing of information that more informed, precise and holistic interventions can be devised and continually tracked, using our performance analysis technologies.

References

Balague, N., Torrents, C., Hristovski, R., & Kelso, J.A.S. (2016). Sport science integration: An evolutionary synthesis. *European Journal of Sport Science, 17*(1), 51–62.

Buekers, M., Ibáñez-Gijón, J., Morice, A., Rao, G., Mascret, N., Laurin, J., et al. (2016). Interdisciplinary research: A promising approach to investigate elite performance in sports. *Quest, 69*, 1–15.

Burwitz, L., Moore, P.M., & Wilkinson, D.M. (1994). Future directions for performance related sports science research: An interdisciplinary approach. *Journal of Sports Sciences, 12*(1), 93–109.

Engelberg, J. (1995). Integrative study in physiology and medicine: Obstacles on the road to integration. *Integrative Physiological and Behavioral Science, 30*, 265–272.

Gould, D., & Damarjian, N. (1998). Mental skills training in sport. In B. Elliott (Ed.), *Training in sport: Applying sport science* (pp. 69–110). Chichester, UK: Wiley & Sons.

Lozano, P.G.B., Avalos-Ramos, M.A., & Vega-Ramirez, L. (2020). Interdisciplinary experience using technological tools in sport science. *Sustainability, 12*(23), 9840.

Piggott, B., Müller, S., Chivers, P., Papaluca, C., and Hoyne, G. (2018). Is sports science answering the call for interdisciplinary research? A systematic review. *European Journal of Sport Science, 19*, 267–286.

O'Donoghue, P., & Mayes, A. (2013). Performance analysis, feedback and communication in coaching. In T. McGarry, P. O'Donoghue & J. Sampaio (Eds.), *Routledge Handbook of Sports Performance Analysis* (pp. 155–164). London: Routledge.

Szabo, S., & Tolnay, P. (2016). Differentiation and integration in sport science, role and task of interdisciplinary sport science. *International Journal of Kinesiology and Sport Science, 13*(2), 17–23.

Williams, S., & Kendall, L. (2007). Perceptions of elite coaches and sports scientists of the research needs for elite coaching practice. *Journal of Sports Sciences, 25*(14), 1577–1586.

Willimczik, K. (1992). Interdisciplinary sport science: a science in search of its identity. In H. Haag, O. Grupe & A. Kirsch (Eds.), *Sport science in Germany* (pp. 7–36). Berlin: Springer.

4

MULTIMEDIA PERFORMANCE PROFILING

Andrew Butterworth

Introduction

Performance profiling offers a truly detailed and intricate overview of performance in real scenarios. Critical to the success of profiling is the collection, manipulation and interpretation of longitudinal data over multiple seasons; without this, any profiles produced would be largely invalid and unreliable. Whilst profiling has already had considerable scholarly activity dedicated to it, much of it is often drowned in jargon and complexity, meaning a lack of applicability to the analysts' practical workflows. This chapter seeks to provide simple definitions of the processes involved in profiling, alongside practical examples to bring the content to life.

Context Is King

Sports performance is neither stable, nor consistent. Each time an activity is undertaken, there are an abundant number of contextual factors that either positively or negatively impact the outcome. These contextual factors and outside influences have a significant impact on a performer's ability to deliver their optimal performance at any given point, under various different circumstances:

> "We never win away from home"
> "We're always poor in the early kick-offs"
> "We're never good enough to play against the big teams"
> "Looks like a warm one today, the game will be slower"

Such questions and statements, whilst often largely coming from journalists or avid fans, are in fact very important to helping us understand the worth and value

DOI: 10.4324/9781003226659-4

of performance profiling. If we do not consider these (and other) contextual factors when analysing the relative strength or weakness of a performance, we might not fully understand the reasons behind performance outcome. Void of context, an analysis of performance is less valuable than one which has carefully considered any outside influences. O'Donoghue (2013) has previously discussed many possible variables that may impact our understanding of performance indicator strength including: match location (Brown et al., 2002; Cianfrone & Zhang, 2006), match importance (Hale, 2004); match status (O'Donoghue & Tenga, 2001; Taylor et al., 2008); and opposition strength (McGarry & Franks, 1994; Taylor et al., 2008). We must therefore fairly consider such factors in assessing the relative strength or weakness of a performance.

Whilst each of the above is researched with regularity and aplomb, let us use perhaps the most researched contextual variable as a detailed example, home advantage. This is where it is expected that teams playing in their familiar home venue will win more than 50% of their matches. For example, in football, where in the men's international game Pollard and Armatas (2017) discovered significant home advantages in World Cup qualifying, in the domestic club game where Goumas (2017) uncovered the role of the away team's distance covered and time zones crossed in strengthening home advantage, and in the women's game, where an average 54% of matches were won by the home team in European domestic leagues (Pollard & Gomez, 2012). Further strengthening the argument of the role home advantage plays, in the delayed 2020 European Championships all four semi-finalists (England, Denmark, Italy and Spain) played all of their group games in their home country, with England going on to reach the final of the tournament having played just one match (a convincing 4–0 win over Ukraine) away from their familiar home venue, Wembley, with which came vociferous home support.

Indeed, the role of fans and the vocal support that they bring in strengthening home advantage, has been researched more in recent times. During the COVID-19 pandemic (a contextual variable in itself), researchers examined the role of fans, or lack of during national lockdowns, in stadiums and the subsequent impact on such home advantage. Studies correlated that without fans in attendance, home advantage did drop, albeit minimally in the majority of cases. In England, Premier League and Championship teams saw a 1.4% drop in home wins, German leagues saw a 1.6% drop off, Spanish domestic teams saw 0.7% less home wins, whilst more significant drops were seen in Danish (17.5%), Greek (18.3%) and Polish (15.8%) leagues (Bryson et al., 2021).

In other sports, the home advantage phenomenon appears to be just as well embedded with a mass of studies having researched into the prevalence of home advantage, discovering an average 62% home advantage in handball (Lago-Penas et al., 2013); 61% in rugby union (Garcia et al., 2013); 58% in volleyball (Alexandros et al., 2012) and 56% in NHL hockey (Jones, 2009). Such studies into contextual variables unearth an important understanding of each and their potential impact upon the outcome of sporting performance. What they can't do however is predict the prevalence of each, nor how one's own team might respond to that given variable.

This is where performance profiling comes in, helping coaches, staff and performers alike in better understanding the responses and outcomes of each phenomenon, consequently preparing more bespoke tactical plans. Through aggregating longitudinal data sets, creating context-specific performance profiles and examining the strength of results of each, performance analysts can better understand performance.

Profiling in Practice

For example, consider a Premier League football team who throughout a 38-match domestic season will play in 20 different venues, at multiple different times of day, against differing strength of opposition, at various altitudes and temperatures, and under multiple match statuses, notwithstanding the importance of individual matches. They will also compete in two domestic cup competitions, and perhaps a European competition too. Each of these additional competitions adds further complexity to the aforementioned variables, alongside new ones in regard to different continents, perception of competition importance and squad rotations. Comprehensive profiling of performance indicators under each of these contextual variables, accumulating and analysing data over each of these multiple contexts will allow the analysts (and subsequently coaches and players) to know more about the potential performance increase or decrease of both themselves, and their opposition, in each contextual situation.

Consider for example Leicester City in the 2021–2022 season. Competing in a standard 38-game Premier League competition, defending their FA Cup triumph from 2021, a second successive season of European football in the Europa League, the League Cup and the one-off Community Shield match all bring about a huge number of different scenarios and contexts. To help the team better understand the potential impact of their own, and opposition performance levels in each of these contexts, performance profiles could be developed.

First, a profile could be developed for all games Leicester City play that season regardless of competition. That profile in itself will inform them of their typical performance level across all contextual variables e.g., kick off times, opponents, locations and temperatures. Then another profile could be created which examines only the home games they play in that season, but again encompassing all other contextual considerations. It is at this point that the team will be able to start making informed considerations; how does the team perform in *all* matches, as opposed to in all *home* matches? What are the differences in values when they play at home? Is there something that they can learn from this and that they need to factor into their pre match preparations?

From here, they can start to become more and more bespoke; creating a profile of home matches against other top six opposition, which in itself, this profile will then help the team's management and sport science staff understand performance levels against their direct rivals for securing European football. Long gone are the days of standard Saturday 3 pm kick offs, and so given the influx and frequency of television matches changing kick off times, the team might then produce profiles for different times, for example a profile of when they play in the early kick off. They could then examine how they perform away from home, on a Thursday, in 6 pm kick offs with temperate climates of over 25°C. And so on, and so on. Every time an additional, or alternative contextual variable is added, it tells the team something else about how historically they have performed in that scenario, which, in turn, helps for future planning. This can be replicated for all opposition teams as well, whereby they can examine how a specific opposition play in certain scenarios, under certain circumstances.

And as yet, we have not even begun to think about creating unit or individual player profiles, each of which carries significant weight in understanding sporting success further. The analysts might create a performance profile of different starting elevens, to ascertain which is statistically the strongest in any given context, or they might want to consider what the strongest back four line up is; profiling can help them understand this. On an individual level, profiles can also be produced, consider perhaps that a profile of Youri Tielemans could be created for games he plays at home on Saturday 3 pm kick offs, examining his performance indicator values in that context, then we might compare those values to when he plays away on a Tuesday at 7:45 pm in sub-zero temperatures in the county of Staffordshire (akin to the cliché). We might also want to create a profile when he plays for his national team, comparing those values when with his Belgian counterparts, to how well he then performs for his club side.

Each profile, and indeed each iteration of each profile that is created, gives us an incredible knowledge base to work from, and learn from. Each of these examples would provide the analysis and coaching team with clear understanding of how the performer delivers under certain conditions. Such information might be invaluable in helping to select starting players, tactics and strategies in different contexts.

Background

The term *performance profiling* is not unique to sports performance analysis, with a form of the tool having been adopted in many different settings including business, commerce and finance. In sport, other sports science disciplines draw upon their own version too, psychologists for example use performance profiling in their work to establish a psychological profile of an athlete, subjectively assessing key criteria to better their understanding of the athletes they are working with. Often, this assessment is done so in tandem with the athletes own subjective interpretation of their relative strengths and weaknesses using the same criteria, to create a 'gap analysis' that stimulates further conversation, goal setting and intervention. Physical profiles of performance are also created by sports scientists, strength and conditioning coaches and physiotherapists. Here, objective data from testing protocols can be used to build an objective and informed outline of an athlete's characteristics, highlighting areas of strength, and of concern for intervention. In performance analysis, profiling is often misinterpreted and definitions are less clear. A simple search of academic research on the key term produces multiple different definitions, with no clear consensus. Some include subjective data, some physical, some coach perceptions and some athlete perceptions to name but a few.

A Clear and Unambiguous Definition

In the context of performance analysis, a performance profile is a collection of quantitative performance indicator data bought together and presented to the end user in a single output, seamlessly integrated with associated multimedia and considerate of outside constraints. Each profile produced should represent how a subject (individual athlete, unit, team, etc.) performs under certain contextual conditions (e.g. in games only away from home) through displaying objective calculations. There are then two sub-categories to the type of profile that we can create, either a typical performance profile, or a single match performance profile.

Typical Performance Profiles

A typical performance profile calculates data which illustrates a subjects *typical* performance level, and their *variability in performance* over multiple matches. Having collected data over a number of performances, typical performance level is an average (usually using mean or median) to show how that subject performs under those circumstances on a *typical* day, having combined and then averaged the sum. For example, if we collect data from a netball match on the percentage of centre passes that lead to a goal from six matches, we might get figures of 58%, 64%, 57%, 69%, 68% and 77%. If we were to then average these out, we get to a figure of 66% CP2G in a *typical* match.

In some research (e.g. Hughes et al., 2001), this typical has been referred to as a *normal* figure, which suggests that there is some point at which when we add the different matches together, the average figure starts to plateau, giving us a so-called normal value for that indicator that indicates consistency. Suggestions have been made that a measure for that might be within 5% of the mean, though this is hugely problematic, and indicates that all performance indicators should stabilise and eventually normalise, no matter how many matches worth of data that might take. But of course, in reality that is not, and should not be the case; it suggests that this stabilisation, consistency and waiting for normal values to appear is a good thing. But there is no such thing as a normal or stable match, nor a normal indicator. The beauty and excitement of sport is in its unpredictability, its dynamism and its volatility. Sport would be a much weaker product, a boring and predictable one, if we knew exactly the outcome and how that outcome would be reached. In sport, consistency is talked about as a desired product in many cases, and that is true of the final result of the match if our team are going to win a title or trophy. But for each individual indicator we don't want to wait for normality or this artificial stability to form; we just want to know the characteristics of each indicator, be that consistent or inconsistent.

Meanwhile, variability in performance showcases how consistently they achieve that typical figure in each match; do the team consistently score 66% each game, or does it *vary* extensively from match to match, achieving 80% in some games, compared to just 43% in others?

Let's go back to our centre pass to goal figures and acknowledge that there are extremities of 57% and 77%, a range of 20%, this is the variability in performance. We would likely call this team inconsistent, given the rather large spread of values. For this indicator, we'd like to see the typical value be regularly high, and the variability in performance low; e.g. the team consistently produces a high value for this indicator. That isn't the case for all indicators though; we do not want our number of errors to be high, we in fact want the opposite where our errors are typically low in matches. For some indicators meanwhile, we might not want to be consistent and become in fact too predictable to the point where the opposition can pre-plan for this. We must therefore be cognisant of this and recognise that some performance indicators will have values that we want to be consistently high, whilst others we want consistently low. There might be others that we want to be inconsistent, and others that we want to be exceptionally consistent regardless.

Single Match Performance Profiles

Post-match conversations both internally and externally, amongst fans and media, will turn to a question of how well their team performed today. Seeking to understand what they have just seen, those interested will strike up and consider conversations about how good a game it was, or who played well and who played badly. Typically, these conversations are riddled with bias and subjectivity, just like the awarding of 'player of the match' awards which are more than a little contentious at times. Whilst externally amongst fans and the media this will undoubtedly continue, internally for coaching teams, single match performance profiling offers a solution to reliably and quickly interpret the actual strength of a performance.

Single match performance profiles utilise typical match data, alongside the raw data from a single performance, to interpret how good a performance it actually was, compared to what that team typically produces, considering the strength of opposition faced and other contextual variables where desired. Here, we combine our knowledge of typical profiles, with the raw figures from a single performance. First taking the earlier created typical performance data, we then map on the raw figures from a single performance of interest, to see how well we performed in that single match, compared to our typical level. For example, our netball team might achieve 84% in their next game for centre pass to goal. We can take this actual figure they achieved in that one match, and directly overlay it onto the typical data to assess how good this single game was, compared to the typical data. This then gives us an excellent indication of how well the team actually played in this single match, using objective data, not subjective interpretations of "I think we played well today". This can be repeated for multiple indicators together, to create an overall interpretation of how good a game was, in addition to indicator-by-indicator interpretations too.

Prevalence and Use

Profiling is underused, and all too often misunderstood. Existing definitions and techniques, written largely by researchers, have often failed to fully understand the complexity and contextual intricacies, whilst also not fully appreciating or considering the end-users. And whilst some have developed their techniques in empirical contexts with real performance data, the majority have done so with third party data and so the applicability to practice and real-world analysis workflows is missing. Sometimes overly complicated language, lengthy explanations or seemingly complex calculations methods may have unintentionally put off those who might benefit from their use within their daily workflows. Therefore, up until now, the existing techniques have largely failed to make it out of the text book and into practical analysis workflows for the betterment of performance, with the work failing to cross the often all too large chasm between performance analysis research and practical implementation.

Since its early adoption into practical performance analysis workflows by boxing (Butler, 1989), performance profiling has had several different methods and techniques proposed in the research in order to assist in the valid creation of profiles. Underlying all of the techniques is the valid and reliable selection and collection of performance data, critical to any performance analysis system. Then, profiling suggestions have attempted to interpret those performance indicator values within the confines of their environment (e.g. O'Donoghue et al., 2008; O'Donoghue & Cullinane, 2011). However, both of these techniques failed to fully consider how they might combine indicators into a single medium, providing a streamlined experience for the end user. Others (e.g. James et al., 2005; O'Donoghue, 2005) did combine indicators into a single medium with more attention paid to those who might use them, and so are recognised and accepted as the two most conventional methods of performance profiling in recent reviews (Butterworth et al., 2013; O'Donoghue, 2013).

Those review papers summarised suggestions for future profiling techniques, with the former (Butterworth et al., 2013) doing so in the context of sports coaching, an important step forward in contextualising the use of profiling in practical work amongst the coaching process. Thirteen key criteria for future profiling techniques were suggested by that review paper, intended to help researchers and practitioners alike create new and innovative profiling methodologies for use in their work. Here, we'll not discuss those in turn, but instead demonstrate and display a new impactful method for profiling which encompasses all of those.

Developing a Performance Profiling Method

Profiling can be undertaken with any sport, regardless of its team or individual nature, reach or stature. To illustrate the method here, examples from the team sport of netball will be utilised, drawing upon the authors' vast experience in the sport to show the development of profiles for teams, and individuals. Though modelled here in netball, the underlying principles and techniques are generalisable and can be applied to any sport, be it team or individual.

When starting to consider the build of profiles, we must first consider a *what* and a *why* – *What* are we trying to find out? *Why* is this piece of analysis so vital? These questions are true of any performance analysis work, with the same applying to performance profiling, requiring coaches, analysts and in some cases players, to carefully consider *why* profiling is required and *what* they seek to find out via using the methodology. Performance profiles should not be built without a purpose in mind, nor should they be utilised to the extent where they lose meaning and impact. *What* questions might include knowing the strongest starting players, performance levels after long travel, impact of game start time or impact of match importance, to name but a few.

Performance Indicator Selection

Once there has been purpose carefully designated for the creation of profiles, the selection of reliably sourced and coded technical and tactical performance indicators is critical. In all prior techniques, this is a mainstay, with Butterworth et al. (2013) noting that the selection of indicators is pivotal to performance analysis in general, but specifically profiling. Content validity as it is otherwise known is important to ensure that the outputs of all analysis work and all profiles are helping to answer the important questions that coaches have. Of course, if the wrong indicators are selected, then they may not be able to do this. The purpose of this section is not to review the existing literature or practical methods of selecting indicators, but instead to highlight the importance of selecting the correct variables to ensure validity in profiling and be able to answer the desired performance questions.

To ensure that content validity can be attained within the profiles, practitioners might seek to refer back and seek reference from influential academic research in the field (e.g. Hughes & Bartlett, 2002) which has sought to provide guidance and rationalise the choice of indicators for performance analysis systems. Others have also provided suggestions for how this might be achieved through data reduction techniques such as principle components analysis (O'Donoghue, 2008), or determinants of success and the most important indicators in various sports including cricket (Najdan et al., 2014), football (Lepschy et al., 2020) and volleyball (Castro & Mequista, 2010). Such research is valuable in helping determine the indicators which discriminate between winning and losing teams, and so helps in the selection of performance indicators which may provide a bigger impact.

Nuances in the selection of indicators will and should always remain though and statistically driven methods should form only part of the selection process. In deciding upon the final indicators, teams should carefully consider what is most important to them, those which have a statistical significance, and those which align and help understand both the coaching and playing philosophy of the management team.

Collection and Calculation

Data entered into performance profiles can be collected by multiple sources depending on the type of data desired. For tactical data, many will choose to code this data themselves, attaining closely to the coaching and playing philosophies of the team and trying to ensure enhanced reliability. For many sports, this is the only way that data can be collected, with the analyst themselves the data collection mechanic, either completing their coding post-match or live-in match if their skills, and technology, allow. In elite football (and others), the shift is moving very much away from the analysts themselves coding, and instead a reliance on external data companies to do so. This changing landscape of the performance analyst's role, and is also important to be aware of in this context. Third-party data providers now deliver near instantaneous streams of data live during performances as they progress, which opens up opportunity for profiling to be completed and impact upon performance in a more real-time environment.

Technical or physical data might also form part of the data collection for profiling, if that is desired in answering the *what* and *why*. Sophisticated GPS units which collect and store physical metrics, are being used more and more frequently, especially in training environments. The data from these that can be extracted is vast and provides a details dive into the physical metrics that characterise performance at all levels. When correlated with tactical data, this uncovers some exciting new prospects for collaborative analysis and holistic profiling. Though, however the data is ultimately collected, it can then be transformed and manipulated into methodologically sound profiles using simpler than you might think methods to do so.

Creating Typical Performance Profiles

Using a spreadsheet software to create our profiles, we capture the typical performance using the median as a central tendency, and the interquartile range (IQR) for variability in performance. First, for each indicator, we calculate the median of the data set, recommended by O'Donoghue (2013) as a better central marker than the mean, which allows us to ascertain the centre of the data set providing the typical figure. In our sheet, we use the very simple formulae;

=MEDIAN(*Data Range*)

In our running netball example, this would be 66%. The interquartile range, that is the middle 50% of values in a data set ranging from the lower 25th to upper 75th, and shows us how consistent the team is, which in our running example would be from 60% (lower quartile) to 69% (upper quartile, a range of 9). To calculate this, for the lower quartile we use the following formulae;

=PERCENTILE(*Data Range*, 25%)

And for the upper quartile;

=PERCENTILE(*Data Range*, 75%)

where *Data Range* is your full set of data, this provides us the calculations to know our typical performance for this indicator. This, repeated for each indicator, in turn, can then be displayed together in a single profile which encompasses all indicators. Often this will be presented via a radar chart, which naturally lends itself to this kind of data, though the same data can be presented in other charts too (e.g. stacked bar), examples of both of these can be seen in Figures 4.1 and 4.2 which illustrate profiling outputs from a netball data set, using multiple possession based indicators. The choice of chart should be carefully chosen to meet with the needs of the end user. It is also imperative to consider the range of values that might be needed in that one chart too. For example, if profiling tennis, then there are some indicators that will have very low values e.g. number of double faults, which might be in single figures, as opposed to some indicators which will have very high values e.g. first serve speed which may be in excess of 180 km/h. Presented on the same graphic, this will skew the look of the data and cause problems for the interpretation, as O'Donoghue (2013) explained. And so, we must be mindful of this in deciding which profiling output to use, but also in deciding upon our final presentation method for the data we have generated.

Interpretation

It is very important to understand how to interpret these figures and graphics, carefully assessing the typical performance, alongside variability in performance. The smaller the IQR and the closer together the LQ and UQ are, the more consistent a team is, the larger the gap between them, the more inconsistent they are. So, if we compare the figures represented in Figures 4.1 and 4.2, we see that our teams CP2S is consistent and high, while the LTO2G and RTO2G

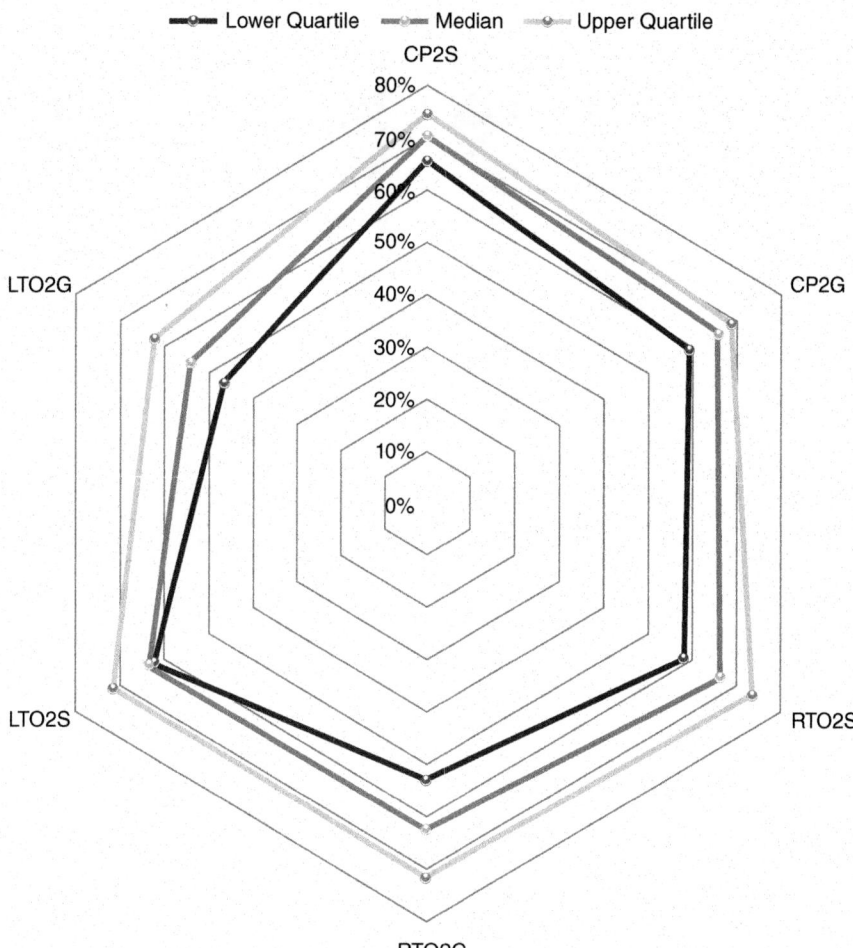

FIGURE 4.1 Typical performance profile (Radar).

are inconsistent. For the indicators presented in these charts, we want to be consistently high on all, since they are attacking variables. However, for others, we
might want to be consistently low (e.g. defensive variables) and for others (e.g.
possession) we might want, need or be forced to be inconsistent. The coaching
expertise, sport knowledge and consideration of each of these figures is therefore
vital for the end product of profiling to be impactful in practice.

This interpretation and understanding of each indicator, in turn, compared
and contrasted is where the value of profiling comes into its own. When we
replicate this process and create a profile for each contextual scenario, we might
be interested in, as per the introduction to this chapter. With a volume of data,

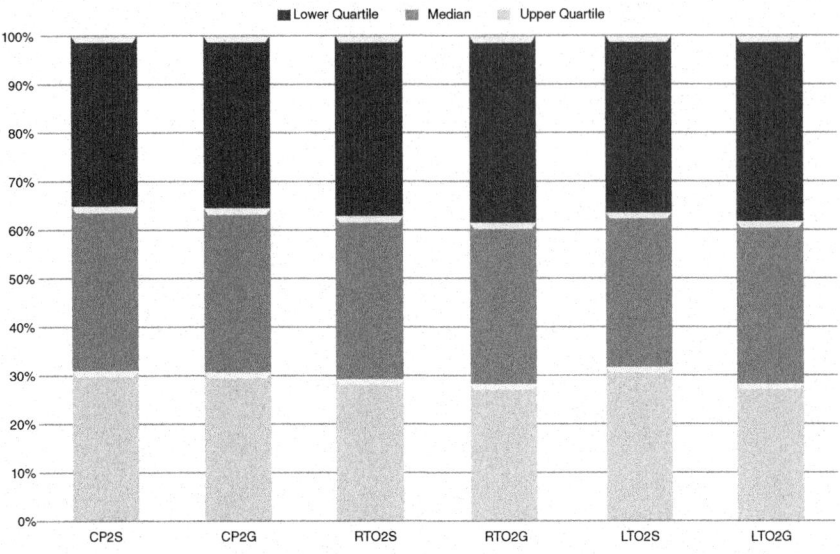

FIGURE 4.2 Typical performance profile (Stacked Bar).

we can easily replicate the process to create profiles for the same indicators in home games, away games, late kick offs, early kick offs, warm weather, cold weather etc. In doing this, we can also start making informed comparisons be-tween individual players typical and IQR figures, or compare the figures of in certain contextual circumstances. We can now compare individuals in the same position vying for a starting spot via directly comparing them to each other. We could use rank formulae within our workbook software to order performers based upon their typical performance level and output a final position for each too. For example, having collected typical data for all athletes of interest, we can directly compare them on each indicator to establish who is best on each and also compare them overall to see who comes out as statistically the strongest player in each position in a squad. This was successful in empirical use during the 2015 Netball World Cup. There, working for England Netball, the system was created to understand and predict opposition starting seven members, so that better tactical plans for counteracting them could be produced. Figure 4.3 is a macroscopic view of all of the rankings of each opposition Australia player, in turn, which led to a final predicted starting seven. Figure 4.4 meanwhile is a closer view of just one of those indicators, outputting the top ranked players in that particular indicator. This model was fully accurate for the nations of New Zealand and Jamaica, whilst for Australia, the seven was impacted by injury, where the first ranked wing attack (WA) was unable to play, with the second placed WA instead starting in the tournament, again confirming its excellent ecological validity.

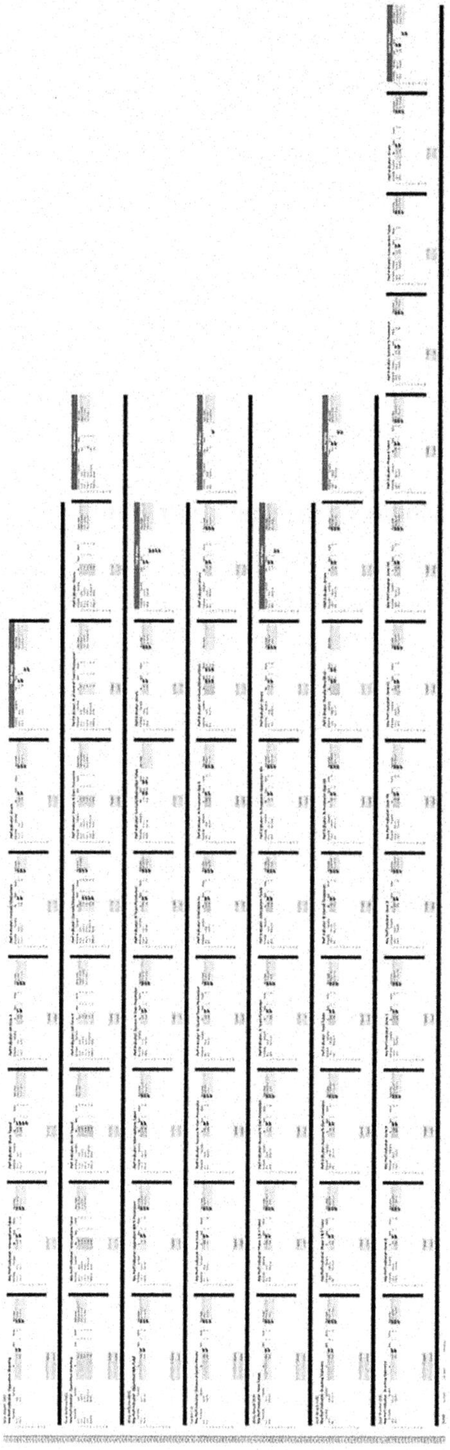

FIGURE 4.3 Macroscopic view of ranking sheet.

Goal Defence (GD)

Key Perf Indicator: Opposition Shooting

	Forename	Surname	%	Rank	Points	Rank Order
1	Laura	Geitz	83%	4	7	Clare McMeniman
2	Julie	Corletto	80%	3	8	Rebecca Bulley
3	Sharni	Layton	84%	5	6	Julie Corletto
4	Clare	McMeniman	75%	1	10	
5	Rebecca	Bulley	78%	2	9	
6						
7						
8						
9						
10						
			86.00%			
			85.00%			

FIGURE 4.4 Detailed view of single ranking indicator.

Creating Single Match Performance Profiles

Single match profiling provides an objective understanding of one match using typical data combined with raw single match data to provide an accurate objective representation of how well the team or athlete actually performed, compared to typical data levels. To create these, we could just take the raw data from a single match, and map those numbers against our already created typical data. Wherever the single match data bands onto within the typical data and IQR, gives us a fair indication of how good the performance was. If the raw data for the single game is higher than the UQ, then it suggests that the team performed well on that indicator, within the top 25% of all performances, if by contrast it sits below the LQ figure, then it might be classed a poor performance, in the lowest 25% of performances. Each indicator can be interpreted and a picture built of how good the game performance was, but also the specific areas individually, that built towards that overall picture.

However, what is missing from that is any form of consideration paid towards any contextual factors in play that day, perhaps the opposition the team have played that day. For example, if a Premier League football team, Leicester City, play a cup game against lower league opposition of considerably lesser quality, then it is likely that they will simply outplay them and the performance indicator values will look extremely high compared to typical and IQR data (for the sake of argument, we are assuming here that a full strength Leicester City team has been deployed). If they play a team in the top half of the Premier League, or a European opposition who are stronger, their performance indicators values will likely drop and map onto lower bandings, given the strength of opposition faced is much greater. This means that a simple method of mapping raw values from a single match to typical data is not enough and may represent a misinterpretation. Therefore, a method by which to interpret the single match, considering the contextual variable (in our example case, opposition faced), is important.

TABLE 4.1 2021 Netball Superleague table and tier rankings

Position	Team	Played	Won	Lost	Drawn	Goals for	Goals against	Goal difference	Points	Rank
1	Loughborough Lightning	20	17	3	0	1,084	803	281	51	1
2	Manchester Thunder	20	17	3	0	1,096	831	265	51	
3	Team Bath Netball	20	17	3	0	950	747	203	51	
4	Leeds Rhinos	20	12	8	0	884	856	28	36	2
5	Saracens Mavericks	20	11	8	1	882	862	20	34	
6	Strathclyde Sirens	20	10	8	2	824	844	−20	32	
7	Wasps	20	10	9	1	884	804	80	31	
8	London Pulse	20	6	14	0	734	793	−59	18	3
9	Severn Stars	20	4	16	0	734	958	−220	12	
10	Surrey Storm	20	3	17	0	775	970	−195	9	4
11	Celtic Dragons	20	1	19	0	675	1,058	−383	3	

First, we need to establish a means by which to rank the different strengths of team that we might face based upon their recent historical performances, this way we can classify them reliably into a tiered strength of opposition. For league-based sports, the recommended method to do this is by using the current league table positions and splitting the teams by accumulated points, in turn allocating them a tier. This means that when created, we have a number of different possible match types, based upon the tier that we attribute to each team. For example, in the 2021 Netball Superleague Season, the table finished as follows in Table 4.1. Using the accumulated points totals, we can then split the table into four distinct tiers of teams based upon those who accumulated similar points totals, and therefore allocating them into a tier of teams. For example, in our table, we see that Loughborough Lightning are a tier one team, and that Celtic Dragons are a tier four team. When they play each other, considering Loughborough Lightning, that results in a 1 versus 4 match type, and when considering Celtic Dragons, that results in a 4 versus 1 match type. In our split of four tiers, there are therefore 16 different possible match types (e.g. 1 vs 1, 1 vs 2, 1 vs 3, 1 vs 4, 2 vs 1, 2 vs 2, 2 vs 3, 2 vs 4, 3 vs 1, 3 vs 2, 3 vs 3, 3 vs 4, 4 vs 1, 4 vs 2, 4 vs 3, and 4 vs 4).

For international sports, the method we might use is world ranking position, deciding upon suitable split lines to allocate their tiers using accumulated ranking points. Using the WTA tennis rankings as an example, at the end of the US Open in 2021, we could split as follows in Table 4.2 where we have used only the top 30 ranked players. We see from these top 30 that there are five tiers and so there are 20 possible match types.

Both of these methods ensure a valid and reliable means by which to split teams into a tier of strength, based on objective points or ranking. There is no limit to the number of tiers that can be created, and the thresholds set to split

TABLE 4.2 WTA rankings and allocated tiers

Rank	Name	WTA points	Tier
1	Ashleigh Barty	9,076	1
2	Aryna Sabalenka	6,995	2
3	Karolína Plíšková	5,255	
4	Iga Świątek	4,756	3
5	Barbora Krejčíková	4,668	
6	Elina Svitolina	4,276	
7	Garbiñe Muguruza	4,250	
8	Sofia Kenin	4,190	
9	Maria Sakkari	3,870	
10	Belinda Bencic	3,735	
11	Petra Kvitová	3,680	
12	Naomi Osaka	3,326	4
13	Anastasia Pavlyuchenkova	3,245	
14	Ons Jabeur	3,100	
15	Angelique Kerber	3,050	
16	Elena Rybakina	2,983	
17	Simona Halep	2,982	
18	Elise Mertens	2,825	
19	Cori Gauff	2,815	
20	Bianca Andreescu	2,563	5
21	Emma Raducanu	2,558	
22	Anett Kontaveit	2,551	
23	Jennifer Brady	2,525	
24	Jessica Pegula	2,435	
25	Karolína Muchová	2,343	
26	Paula Badosa Gibert	2,298	
27	Danielle Collins	2,260	
28	Leylah Fernandez	2,254	
29	Daria Kasatkina	2,140	
30	Jeļena Ostapenko	2,025	

teams should by dynamic to respond to the ongoing evolving process. For example, all of our tier 1 teams in our Netball Superleague table have 51 points and an exceptionally similar goal difference, and whilst although Leeds Rhinos also qualified for the end of season play offs (and so technically we could class in the same tier), their points and goal difference see them classed as a lower tier team. In our WTA example, we see that Ashleigh Bartey has a significantly higher number of points than Aryna Sabalenka ranked second, and so a separate tier is created. This allocation of tiers is an ongoing and dynamic process by which analysts and coaches should carefully discuss the ranking they are going to attribute to each team or individual, justifying that via the points accumulated or ranking points. These will need updating as changes are made and the bandings potentially shift for different teams and athletes.

Once tiers and match types are established, our next step is to create typical data sets for each possible match type. We therefore create a typical data set for each of our earlier mentioned 20 matches that could take place. To do this, we utilise a split of quintiles to create our typical data set, which creates five equally distributed sets of data, 0–20, 21–40, 41–60, 61–80 and 81–100. Each of these bands represents and aggregates the typical figure expected for each indicator, based upon the number of performances that fall into that range. This ensures that when we interpret our single match raw data later on, we can do so in a clear manner and provide accurate descriptive explanations of how good the single match really was. To this end, in our workbook, we use the following for each of those bandings;

=PERCENTILE(*Data Range*, 20%)
=PERCENTILE(*Data Range*, 40%)
=PERCENTILE(*Data Range*, 60%)
=PERCENTILE(*Data Range*, 80%)

These are used for each indicator, each time selecting the data range for matches only played under that match type and reported back in a table of all values. Table 4.3 illustrates this in practice, with elite netball data represented when a tier one team plays against others of different strengths.

With such typical data sets established for each indicator under each possible match type, we can now accurately interpret a single match worth of data, and objectively ascertain how strong it really was, considering the strength of opposition faced. Having created this data set, the interpretation is simple, by establishing

TABLE 4.3 Netball match type norms

Match type	Quintile banding	CP2S	CP2G	RTO2S	RTO2G	LTO2S	LTO2G
1 vs 1	20%	67%	57%	58%	51%	56%	47%
	40%	71%	63%	68%	61%	62%	54%
	60%	74%	67%	75%	70%	70%	61%
	80%	80%	71%	82%	75%	85%	81%
1 vs 2	20%	69%	64%	67%	62%	60%	57%
	40%	73%	68%	71%	71%	68%	65%
	60%	78%	70%	76%	75%	74%	73%
	80%	82%	73%	83%	81%	85%	83%
1 vs 3	20%	71%	68%	72%	69%	72%	67%
	40%	74%	70%	78%	73%	78%	73%
	60%	77%	71%	81%	77%	83%	77%
	80%	83%	73%	85%	83%	86%	82%
1 vs 4	20%	72%	66%	64%	60%	79%	75%
	40%	77%	68%	65%	63%	82%	78%
	60%	81%	71%	72%	72%	85%	82%
	80%	84%	75%	86%	86%	88%	85%

TABLE 4.4 Descriptive data interpretation bandings

Quintile banding	Descriptor
0–20	Very poor
21–40	Poor
41–60	Average
61–80	Good
81–100	Very good

between which of our quintiles the single match figures fall. Descriptive interpretations of this can be provided, using recommendations as per Table 4.4.

For example when a tier one team play another tier one team in our Table 4.3 example, if they take 80% or more of their centre passes to a shot (CP2S), this is in the top 20% of all netball performances for this match type and classed as very good, whilst if they were to take between 71% and 74% this would be average, and less than 67% would be classed as very poor. We now take the final raw performance indicator values from a single match of interest, and map these onto our earlier established match type norms. Once again, we might consider presenting this via a radar chat, as in the example of a 2 versus 1 match type in elite netball (Figure 4.5). The hatched line (which is also usually coloured red, though not displayed in this figure image due to formatting) is the raw data from the single match of interest, and the black lines typical performance using one of our new quintile norms set.

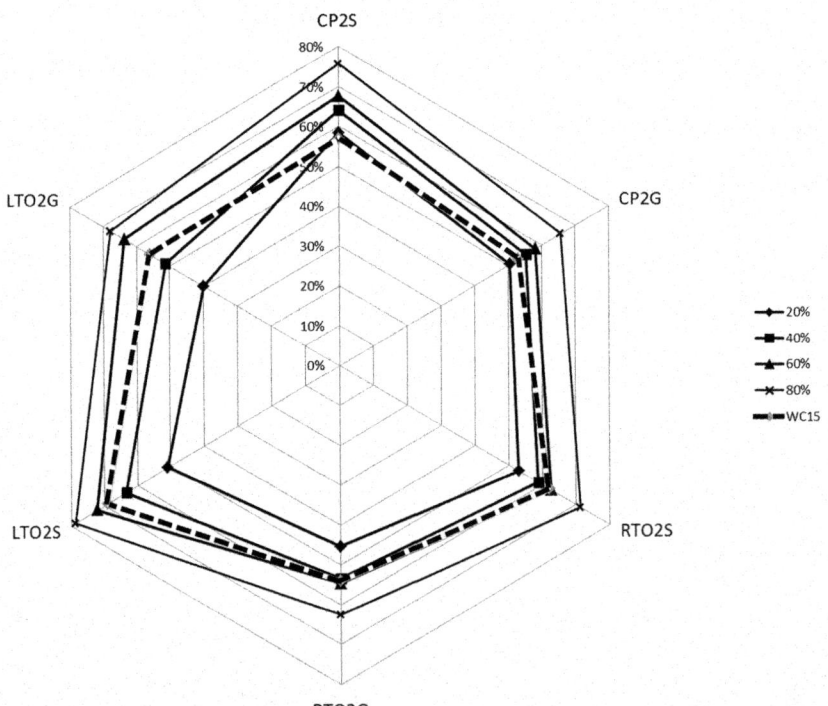

FIGURE 4.5 2 vs. 1 single match profile.

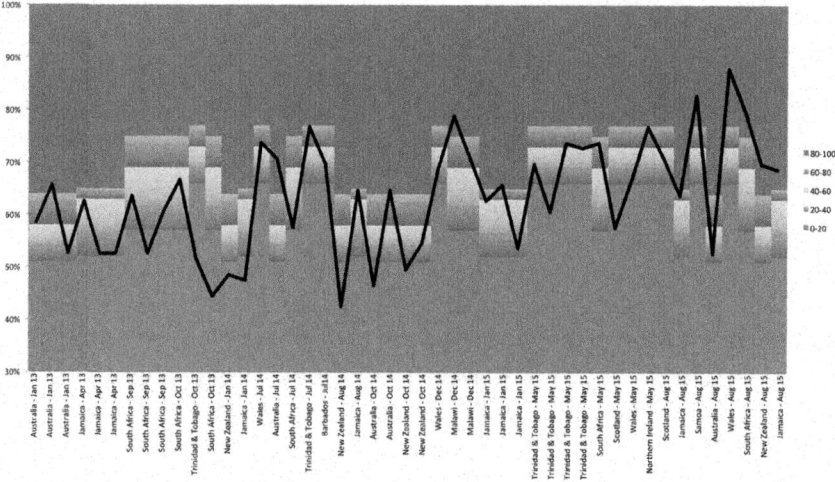

FIGURE 4.6 Longitudinal trend analysis.

In Figure 4.5, we therefore learn that this single performance saw a very poor performance for CP2S, a poor performance on CP2G and average performances on all remaining indicators. This method allows us to establish the strength of each performance indicator in turn, showing areas of strength and weakness in the single match being analysed, this offers an excellent means by which to identify areas to work on and bring back into the coaching process for further attention. To track fluctuations in performance over time, we might also consider placing each individual match on a continuum, tracking consistency match-to-match. This can be achieved by placing the typical data (split into quintiles) in the background, with a trend line for the raw data of each individual fixture, allowing us to track the indicator over time. An example here (Figure 4.6) of a netball teams' performance on a single indicator establishes their inconsistencies over a multi-year period.

Profile Presentation

Having moved forward with valid and reliable calculations of profiling data for both typical and single performances, considerable deliberation is still required as to the presentation of such profiles back into the coaching process. If we were to present back our tables and radar charts, this would likely overwhelm and confuse our end users. If we are looking to present just the data, but in a more attractive manner then we might make use of new and evolving technologies, such as those explored in Chapter 2, which offer considerable promise for streamlining the data delivery. Specific data visualisation software such as Tableau, Microsoft PowerBI or Sisense provide an opportunity to deliver interactive and attractive visualisations to bring this profiling data to life. However, these still offer only the data in numerical format and so are still void of context and interactivity, seen as key recommendations for future profiling techniques in those critical review papers (e.g. Butterworth et al., 2013). And so, we must consider how we bring these figures to life, in context and with associated multimedia evidence, which is a critical learning aid.

Before that though, if we start to present our profiles talking about typical performance, match types, single match profiling, interquartile range, ranking or predicted teams, we'll likely lose our audience before we even have them. So, the first thing we consider is the language used, suggesting here that we refer to typical performance as *average*, a term that coaches and athletes are much more familiar with and does not lose its meaning in our true understanding of the methodology. The upper quartile we refer to as *best performances*, and the lower as *worst performances*, which help end users to understand the context of what they are looking at and the interpretation of it in simple language. With the IQR being represented in this manner, end users can understand the difference between them on a good day, e.g. what they are capable of at their best, on a bad day, and what they do on average.

Presenting the profiling data alongside associated multimedia needs to be done inside specialist software and might be considered in presentation software such as PowerPoint, Keynote or Prezi, each of which allow data from profiling, alongside carefully selected multimedia to be presented congruently. We must of course be careful not to overwhelm our end users though, and so a maximum of six to eight clips are recommended, which should be no older than six months or ten performances. Figure 4.7 illustrates an example of such a multimedia profile completed for use by a single athlete in badminton (anonymity protected via removing athlete picture and name). Versions of each profile would need to be made for each end user, e.g. the team as a whole, units, individual players etc. Templates for each would be helpful for this before data are manually transferred

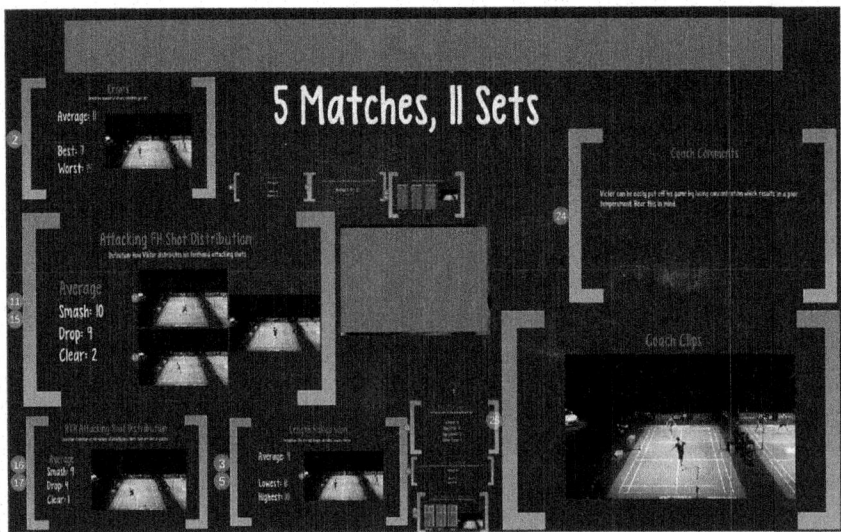

FIGURE 4.7 Multimedia performance profile.

into the individual profile as updates are required. These interactive end products then allow a more meaningful and deeper learning process to occur.

Though what we have just described is a somewhat time consuming and laborious process which would involve the analyst exporting video out of their analysis software and into the presentation medium, combining with the profiling data on a regular basis to ensure it is updated. We can streamline this process further by creating our multimedia profiles in output window software contained within our analysis packages. Scripting in Hudl SportsCode can be used for this purpose which will allow profiling data represented via databases to be combined with the correct video clips, whilst in Catapult Pro Video – Focus or NacSport, we can also use their output window and graphic features too to create interactive profiling outputs.

Implementation and Use in the Coaching Process

Multimedia performance profiles provide ample opportunity to impact on practice. Serving multiple purposes within the dynamic coaching process, profiles can have significant impact on the role of analysis and the outcome of performance. Here, some of the key areas in which profiling might be useful are considered in turn.

Selection

The selection of players for squads or upcoming matches is critical, a decision which usually falls to a head coach or manager. Not only does the decision on who to select impact upon the outcome of the match itself, but also wider repercussions for athlete and coaches' careers too (Fiander et al., 2021). Satisfaction, wellbeing and enjoyment are said to be linked with participation in sport for athletes, whilst for coaches it presents a valuable opportunity to reflect on action, critically appraising the selection decisions that they did make (Downham & Cushion, 2020). Traditionally, selection to squads or starting positions is a process undertaken by coaches or selectors, which by its human nature precludes objectivity. Resultantly, most selections are biased, subjective and open to interpretation. Empirical research tends to agree, with Bradbury and Forsyth (2012) suggesting that subjective selection decisions, characterised by unclear or unspecified selection criteria, can lead to controversy and debate. This debate might come anecdotally by fans and the media pre-game, or internally within clubs via players, staff and coaches questioning decisions and internal processes. Whilst the former is undesirable, the latter is perhaps more serious, especially since there are potential repercussions.

Bradbury and Forsyth's (2012) research explains that selection decisions (and any associated controversy) might not only impact upon current sporting involvements and playing time satisfaction, but in the wider context of their lives too including sponsorship, image rights, endorsement and other income opportunities. Elsewhere, Fiander et al.'s (2021) research reports that deselection might be associated with stress, crisis, identity loss and a feeling of redundancy. Ethics too are considered a problem, with research (e.g. Collins et al., 1999) indicating that there is the potential for professional and legal conflicts unless objectivity is improved. It is then still surprising that there is so little objectivity seemingly associated with selection and an apparent lack of data or impartiality used for selection decisions in the majority of environments.

That said, in some sports, data and a form of profiling is used, and since suggestions were made that further objectivity was required in selection decisions, significant progress has been made. In baseball, Fritz and Bukiet (2010) sought to provide objectivity in ranking players, though their primary objective was to determine the MVP, rather than inform selection. In cricket, the use of performance analysis, more specifically data and a form of profiling, is already well embedded and critical to the coaching process and selection decisions. Practically, cricket is known as a sport which regularly uses reliable data collection mechanisms, whilst there is also a growing body of practical academic research too. For example, Sharma et al. (2012) offer a novel method for the ordering and selection of T20 batsmen, based upon ordered weighting averages which was modelled in the Indian Premier League competition. Amin and Sharma (2014) popularised a model for the for selection of players via data envelopment analysis, ensuring vital objectivity for selection, meanwhile Saikia et al. (2016) suggested a model for the selection of all positions in cricket, also noting that this could be extended to other sports too. At the moment though, this seems rare and as yet unembedded in frequent practice, with Fiander et al. (2021) reviewing the sport coaching literature and establishing that for most, subjective measures such as intuition, mentality, behaviour and experience are still the basis of selection decisions.

And so, as sport and performance analysis seek to move forwards, with data playing more and more of a pivotal role in that, there is a strong case for increasing objectivity and using data to do so. Building performance profiles of teams, units and athletes (considerate of context) offers a genuine opportunity to drive practice forwards, increase professionalism and attend to some of our earlier concerns regarding current practice. Each profile, coupled with the ranking and ordering methods proposed earlier in this chapter, offers a promising step forward in increasing objectivity amongst selection decisions. Where adopted, these profiles can provide objectivity based upon real, historical data, and so should they wish to utilise it, this can help inform coaches and selectors, attaining to any concerns or controversies regarding their decisions.

Opposition Analysis

During pre-match analysis in the lead up to a game day, analysts will traditionally spend considerable time assessing the opposition, seeking to unearth some key trends that their own athletes should be aware of. Usually, this is predominantly dominated by video analysis and subjective analysis work which seeks to find patterns from what the analyst sees, or thinks they see. Data though is becoming more and more involved in opposition and pre-match analysis, as analysts seek to enhance the reliability and objectivity in their work. Highlighted in Chapter 2, the number of data companies readily available streams now available is growing, with near automation for many. This opens up an opportunity to utilise that data (or data generated by the analysts own coding) in profiles to help better understand the particular nuances of play that might emerge in the next match.

Using the player comparison tool shown in this chapter provides a means by which to predict starting members of the team, and allows for a more detailed tactical plan to be built around those players. If used, the profiles created hold promise in enabling coaches to have a better understanding of what they might see and seek to annul their strengths, whilst exploiting their weaknesses. This of course in turn ensures that players are better prepared and have clear strategies in place for the matches ahead. In their recent 2021 Netball Superleague season, the victorious championship winning side Loughborough Lightning utilised profiling extensively to this end, and planned in great detail for key individual players. Such plans played out in reality and the team were able to utilise the analysis performed in order to nullify opposition strengths. This work was in part credited as a success factor in the win with advocates soon becoming apparent in the media and in coaching circles.

Target Setting

The use of target setting in the sport sciences is commonplace, with multiple disciplines seeking to offer athletes a parameter that they should aspire to reach. In physical sciences that might be a new lowest time for a distance covered, or a new personal best in the gym. For performance analysis, we often see analysts or coaches providing their athletes with an aim of reaching a higher target for a technical or tactical skill, maybe increasing their netball shooting percentage to 93%. Further, in existing models of performance analysis and the coaching process, target setting is often a core element, with Horne's (2013) model in particular a central example of this, which has a constant setting and evolution of targets as a fundamental part of the model.

What is less commonly discussed or known is how these targets are set and if there is in fact any science behind them. Furthermore, how to reach those targets, how long it might take or how an athlete knows if they have reached those levels are also commonly missing. Performance profiling, especially typical profiling, offers a means by which to develop more objectivity to this process and help answer those questions. Through tracking variability and consistency in performance over time using typical profiling, in tandem with individual single match profiles, the objectivity that can be added can be a core driver of target setting conversations. Fluctuations in performance over time can be accurately traced which leads to accurate insights into the levels needed to reach peak performance. Modelling profiles also offers the opportunity to help deliver an insight into how long it might take to reach the target, based upon incremental increases over time. Of course, this then impacts upon the training of technical and tactical skills in practice, which can aid in coaching plans and long-term athlete development planning.

Talent ID/Recruitment

If profiles are used with young athletes developing through their skill, maturation and socio-cognitive development stages, they might prove an exceptionally value tool for talent ID and recruitment analysts in sport. Where profiles are built from a young age, the trend analysis and typical performance monitoring allows ample opportunity for the tracking of progression or regression over time for individual indicators, but also overall performance level. This insight can be highly valuable in the development of young players coming through, and helping them (and their coaches) understand their current position, and those areas that they need to develop further. A form of gap analysis can be utilised to ascertain where the young player is currently, and where they need to get to in order to reach similar levels. Again, time is crucial to this and so tracking these fluctuations consistently over time is vital to ensure that a valid and reliable measure of performance development can be ascertained. Equally though, the implementation of profiles must be done carefully and with great caution to ensure that the enjoyment, fun and passion is not sucked from young athletes who could lose their will, desire and freedom to play and develop. If the focus is becoming too heavily set on performance indicators and set targets, coaches and analysts might consider creative ways to relax their young athletes and ensure their freedom to develop is not overshadowed by pressures from data driven sources.

For recruitment analysts, using the large swathes of external data often available in many sports in profiling methods will also offer an opportunity to see those players who for the mould, holding the particular attributes required for the team. Analysts will be able to build valid and reliable profiles of athletes under different circumstances and contexts, to better understand if they fit the playing model and philosophies of the club.

Post-match

As a match finishes, template-based profiling means that analysts can produce valid and reliable indications of match strengths in short time periods. Using the methods of profiling outlined in this chapter, analysts are able to attribute objectivity and accurately rank how good a single performance was. This is a valuable resource that helps quantify and objectify the performance just finished. Traditionally, post-match briefs are dominated by subjective opinions and interpretations of performance, but profiling offers and objective upgrade to that, in near real time, to help deliver better coaching conversations, fully engrained in context.

Concluding Remarks

Multimedia performance profiling offers analysts, coaches and players alike an objective and informed view of performances over longer time periods and single match interpretations, considering contextual influences upon their performance such as the venue, opposition or match surface. Following a thorough review of prior techniques, the method proposed in this chapter offers an easy way to follow practical guide for creating profiles. Used practically in an interactive and collaborative manner with video, photo and audio, multimedia profiles offer a valid and reliable interpretation that can help inform coaching decisions and seek ultimately, to help increase performance levels.

References

Alexandros, L., Panagiotis, K., & Miltiades, K. (2012). The existence of home advantage in volleyball. *International Journal of Performance Analysis in Sport, 12*(2), 272–281.

Amin, G., & Sharma, S. (2014). Cricket team selection using data envelopment analysis. *European Journal of Sport Science, 14*(1), 369–376.

Bradbury, T.M., & Forsyth, D.K. (2012). You're in; you're out: selection practices of coaches. *Sport, Business and Management, 2*(1), 7–20.

Brown, T.D. Jr., Van Raalte, J.L., Brewer, B.W., Winter, C.R. & Cornelius, A.E. (2002). World Cup soccer home advantage. *Journal of Sport Behaviour, 25*(2), 134–144.

Bryson, A., Dolton, P., Reade, J.J., Schreyer, D., & Singleton, C. (2021). Experimental effects of an absent crowd on performances and refereeing decisions during COVID-19. *Institute for the Study of Labor (IZA) Discussion Papers*, No. 13578.

Butler, R.J. (1989). Psychological preparation of Olympic boxers. In J. Kremer & W. Crawford (Eds.), *The psychology of sport: theory and practice* (pp. 74–84). Belfast: BPS Northern Ireland Branch.

Butterworth, A.D., O'Donoghue, P., & Cropley, B. (2013). Performance profiling in sports coaching: A review. *International Journal of Performance Analysis in Sport, 13*(3), 572–593.

Castro, J.M., & Mesquita, I. (2010). Analysis of the attack tempo determinants in volleyball's complex II – A study on elite male teams. *International Journal of Performance Analysis in Sport, 10*(3), 197–206.

Cianfrone, B.A. & Zhang, J.J. (2006). Differential effects of television commercials, athlete endorsements, and venue signage during a televised action sports event. *Journal of Sport Management, 20*(3), 322–344.

Collins, D., Moore, P., Mitchell, D., & Alpress, F. (1999). Role conflict and confidentiality in multidisciplinary athlete support programmes. *British Journal of Sport Medicine, 33*, 208–211.

Downham, L., & Cushion, C. (2020). Reflection in a high-performance sport coach education program: a foucauldian analysis of coach developers. *International Sport Coaching Journal, 7*(3), 347–359.

Fiander, M., Stebbings, J., Coulson, M., & Phelan, S. (2021). The information coaches use to make team selection decisions: A scoping review and future recommendations. *Sports Coaching Review*, ahead of print. https://doi.org/10.1080/21640629.2021.1952812

Fritz, K., & Bukiet, B. (2010). Objective method for determining the most valuable player in major league baseball. *International Journal of Performance Analysis in Sport, 10*(2), 152–169.

Garcia, M.S., Aguilar, O.G., Lazo, C.J.V., Marques, P.S., & Romero, J.J.F. (2013). Home advantage in home nations, five nations and six nations rugby tournaments (1883–2011). *International Journal of Performance Analysis in Sport, 13*(1), 51–63.

Goumas, C. (2017). Tyranny of distance: Home advantage and travel in international club football. *International Journal of Performance Analysis in Sport, 14*(1), 1–13.

Hale, S.L. (2004). Work-rate of Welsh National League players in training matches and competitive matches. In P. O'Donoghue & M.D. Hughes (Eds.), *Performance analysis of sport VI* (pp. 35–44). Cardiff: CPA, UWIC Press.

Hughes, M., Evans, S., & Wells, J. (2001). Establishing normative profiles in performance analysis. *International Journal of Performance Analysis in Sport, 1*, 4–27.

Hughes, M., & Bartlett, R.M. (2002). The use of performance indicators in performance analysis. *Journal of Sport Sciences, 20*(10), 739–754.

Horne, S. (2013). The role of performance analysis in elite netball competition structures. In D. Peters & P. O'Donoghue (Eds.), *Performance analysis of Sport IX* (pp. 30–37). London: Routledge.

James, N., Mellalieu, S.D., & Jones, N.M.P. (2005). Establishing normative profiles in performance analysis. *Journal of Sport Sciences, 23*, 63–72.

Jones, M.B. (2009). Scoring first and home advantage in the NHL. *International Journal of Performance analysis in Sport, 9*(3), 320–331.

Lago-Penas, C., Gomez, M., Viano, J., Gonzalez-Garcia, I., & Fernandez-Villarino, M. (2013). Home advantage in elite handball: The impact of the quality of opposition on team performance. *International Journal of Performance Analysis in Sport, 13*(3), 724–733.

Lepschy, H., Wasche, H., & Woll, A. (2020). Success factors in football: An analysis of the German Bundesliga. *International Journal of Performance Analysis in Sport, 20*(2), 150–164.

McGarry, T. & Franks, I.M. (1994). A stochastic approach to predicting competition squash match-play. *Journal of Sports Sciences, 12*(6), 573–584.

Najdan, M., Robins, M., & Glazier, P. (2014). Determinants of success in English domestic Twenty20 cricket. *International Journal of Performance Analysis in Sport, 14*(1), 276–295.

O'Donoghue, P. (2008). Principal components analysis in the selection of key performance indicators in sport. *International Journal of Performance Analysis in Sport, 8*(3), 145–155.

O'Donoghue, P., Mayes, A., Edwards, K., & Garland, J. (2008). Performance norms for British superleague netball. *International Journal of Sports Science and Coaching, 3*, 501–511.

O'Donoghue, P. (2013). *Sports performance profiling.* In T. McGarry, P. O'Donoghue, & J. Sampaio (Eds.), *Routledge handbook of sports performance analysis* (pp. 127–139). London: Routledge.

O'Donoghue, P., & Cullinane, A. (2011). A regression based approach to interpreting sports performance. *International Journal of Performance Analysis in Sport, 11*, 295–307.

O'Donoghue, P., & Tenga, A. (2001). The effect of scoreline on work rate in elite soccer. *Journal of Sports Sciences, 19*(1), 25–26.

Pollard, R., & Armatas, V. (2017). Factors affecting home advantage in football World Cup qualification. *International Journal of Performance Analysis in Sport, 17*(1), 121–135.

Pollard, R., & Gomez, M.A. (2012). Comparison of home advantage in men's and women's football leagues in Europe. *International Journal of Performance Analysis in Sport, 14*(1), 77–83.

Saikia, H., Bhattacharjee, D., & Radhakrishnan, U. (2016). A new model for player selection in cricket. *International Journal of Performance Analysis in Sport, 16*(1), 373–388.

Sharma, S.K., Amin, R.G., & Gattoufi, S. (2012). Choosing the best Twetny20 cricket batsmen using ordered weighting average. *International Journal of Performance Analysis in Sport, 12*(3), 614–628.

Taylor, J.B., Mellalieu, S.D., James, N. & Shearer, D. (2008). The influence of match location, qualify of opposition and match status on technical performance in professional association football. *Journal of Sports Science, 26*, 885–895.

5

PERFORMANCE ANALYSIS AS A COACH DEVELOPMENT TOOL

Andrew Butterworth and Jon Woodward

Introduction

The symbiotic relationship between the coaching process and performance analysis is now well documented. This and the impact our discipline also plays in developing processes can further develop coaching practice as a whole. Whilst the interpretation and understanding of coaching practice and associated behaviours is not always easy or always quantifiable, it is incredibly important in the ongoing improvement of coaches. In fact, for any coach, it is vital to take stock and consider their own development through means which might include experience, qualifications or via an impactful and relevant reflective analytical method. Part of that reflective process might be to consider the behaviours that they as a coach exhibit when they are delivering directly to players, or interacting with other staff. This is important as the way in which the coach behaves and conducts themselves has direct impact on others, including on their performance, learning and emotions. Whereas many things in the coaching process are not controllable, these actual behaviours, including the physical actions, words and expressions by a coach, are both controllable and measurable, and critically, changeable.

But to change something in any area of life, there needs to first be a recognition of requirement or desire to do so. Therefore, the coach must be willing to engage (or asked to do so), putting themselves in a slight state of vulnerability, since it is their job which will be under the microscope, and engage with a process that requires humility to provide a better end outcome. Klein (2010) considers that the improvement of performance is to move through a period of errors and uncertainty and attempt to reduce or lessen these. That, coupled with the development of insights to support the process of improvement can lead to evolution or

DOI: 10.4324/9781003226659-5

revolution in a form of change. Those insights for change might be provided by analysis, since the change process will also require evidence and resources in the form of video, audio or data. Here, performance analysis is useful in assisting the facilitation of recording coach behaviours using our advanced technology. Much in the same way we would film and code the sporting actions or behaviours of athletes in training or a match, the skill set is here being applied in a different context. The selection of indicators, recorded sessions and reflective processes that ensue as part of this are all vitally important to the coach being able to make changes.

Pedagogy, Philosophy and Reflection

As soon as you see these words, you, as a performance analyst, might be put off or wondering their applicability to you. Later in this chapter, we are going to discuss in detail the role of performance analysis and the practical requirements of using our discipline as a tool to help coaches. If we are to do that, we have to first know about the areas of practice that are especially important to coaches, heightening our appreciation so that we can become an integral part of their development. This involvement is ever more critical since the role of analysis in aiding coaches is becoming more widespread, with specific parts of analyst positions, or entire roles dedicated towards it.

We discovered earlier in Chapter 1 that the coaching process involves both the coach and the performer having a common understanding of the process which is linked to the athlete's goals, the organisation, and the level of commitment from both groups (Lyle & Cushion, 2017). Coaching is a complex and multifaceted activity which if deemed effective is said to involve the consistent application of integrated professional, interpersonal and intrapersonal knowledge with a view to enhancing performance factors including competence and confidence (Lyle, 2002; Cote & Gilbert, 2009; Jones & Kingston, 2013). There are a number of models available *of* and *for* the coaching process as examined in chapter one of this book which, depending on your view, help guide the coach towards successful practice. Underpinning that practice is the concept of coaching pedagogy, which Watkins and Mortimer (1999) defined as conscious activity by one person designed to enhance learning in another. Developing that pedagogy is critical if a coach is to be effective as described above, and to help athletes towards their end goals. As a key developmental part of this, it is also critical in that the coach is seeking to develop and enhance their own expertise and practice.

Coaching Philosophy

It is essential that the coaching process, along with the application of the coaching pedagogy and the intended outcomes (e.g. participation, talent development or elite performance), is aligned to an underpinning or guiding philosophy (either recognised or assumed). There are a range of varying definitions of what a coaching philosophy is, with Burton and Raedeke (2008) defining coaching philosophy as a set of beliefs and principles that guide your behaviour, allowing each individual coach to be true to their values, whilst Walsh (2009) believes coaching philosophy is a blueprint for action, indicating what, when and why things should be done. Within the sector and more in-depth analysis of coaching and its application, it is acknowledged that having a coaching philosophy is vital to an individual's coaching practice as it provides a set of guiding principles and allows for self-realisation and identification of values held nearest to each individual (Lyle, 2002). Two types of value underpin a coaching philosophy (knowingly or not) and are the guiding principles that influence the actions used by a coach. Terminal values are the end-goal outcomes, e.g. winning a cup competition, whilst instrumental values are the personal behaviours required to achieve that end goal, e.g. honesty, creativity, ambition, innovation and logic. How those values are formed varies hugely coach to coach, but typically are driven by what an individual perceives to be of importance to themselves, their perceptions, prior experiences or their educational, developmental and reflective journeys.

Reflective Practice

Reflective practice is commonly used as a phrase in sport but perhaps not always understood and sometimes seen by reluctant engagers as a mammoth task with little practical end use. If engaged with properly, reflective practice is incredibly valuable, giving guidance and action toward positive improvements in tangible outcomes. Reflective practice is the concept of professionals thinking about what they are doing (reflection in-action), or have done (reflection on-action), and re-think alternative actions or responses in future iterations (Schön, 1983). It has been used extensively in sports coaching previously and also within academic courses too. The importance of reflective practice is further realised when considering it has been found that many coaches work without any reference to a coaching model within their role, as they tend to base their practice on previous experience and events (Cross, 1995; Saury & Durand, 1998; Gilbert & Trudel, 2001; Cushion et al., 2003; Jones et al., 2004). Resultantly, the process of reflection and review by the coach, perhaps with assistance from others, is a key element to utilise in the development of the coaching craft and enhancing end user outcomes.

Several models to aid reflection have been put forwards, including Kolb and David's (2014) cycle of reflection. Within this cycle, it is expected that those engaging with it will 'start' by having an experience, before moving onto subsequent steps to consider the meaning of that, and alternative responses next time. Other models exist too; however, it should be noted that in the wider practical application of coaching, not all coaches consciously follow a process of formal reflection based on models, however, by undertaking a more structured and formal process, the changing influence on actions and outcomes could be accounted for.

Coach Awareness

For any coach to be proficient in their delivery, it is suggested that they must consider a number of areas to fully develop and understand the expertise required which considers the full breadth of the coaching environment(s) in which the coach operates in. By understanding the framework of Abraham et al. (2009), the coach should be able to plan, deliver and review coaching sessions, either as individual sessions, or within an event-, seasonal- or performance-cycle. With these considerations, they can adapt their coaching process application through a series of behaviours and strategies:

1. Understanding the *Athlete* – Movement, Physical and Mental
   – Including Psychological, Social & Personal Psychology, Physiology, Sociology, Biomechanics, Motor Control, Nutrition
2. Understanding the *Sport* – Technique, Tactics, Sport Specific Conditioning and Mental Skills
   – Including Perception, Decision Making, Technical Models
3. Understanding *Pedagogy* – Drills, Practices, Communication, Behaviour
   – Including Situational Learning, Coaching Programmes of Work, Motor Learning, Discovery Learning, Learning Concepts (such as Constructivism and Behaviourism), Coaching Concepts (such as Teaching Games for Understanding), Dynamical Systems
4. Understanding the *Context* – Club, NGB, Sport, Performance Level, Parental Influences
   – Including Policy, Psychology, Sociology
5. Understanding *Self* – Reflective Practice, Self-Critique and -Analysis, Personal Effectiveness
   – Including Beliefs, Assumptions, Attitudes, Critical Thinking, Emotional Intelligence, Excellence Behaviours
6. Understanding *Process and Practice* of Coaching – Problem Solving, Orchestrating, Planning, Reviewing
   – Including Metacognition, Cognitive Psychology, Decision Making, Critical Thinking, Strategic Awareness, Situation Awareness

Building upon this, UK Coaching (formerly known as Sportscoach UK), the organisation who support and help coaches, further considered the concepts in creating their coach learning framework (as seen in Figure 5.1). This framework was developed following a bespoke research project to inform applied practice, which includes the recognition of nine themes. These are important as they help the coach to understand their role more holistically and the important areas that they need to consider when delivering their coaching directly to athletes. UK Coaching also have their own coach development resources to support coaches available on their platform, through which they have further considered the key behaviours that underpin effective coaching practice, broken down into sub-themes of personal, people and practice (Figures 5.2 and 5.3).

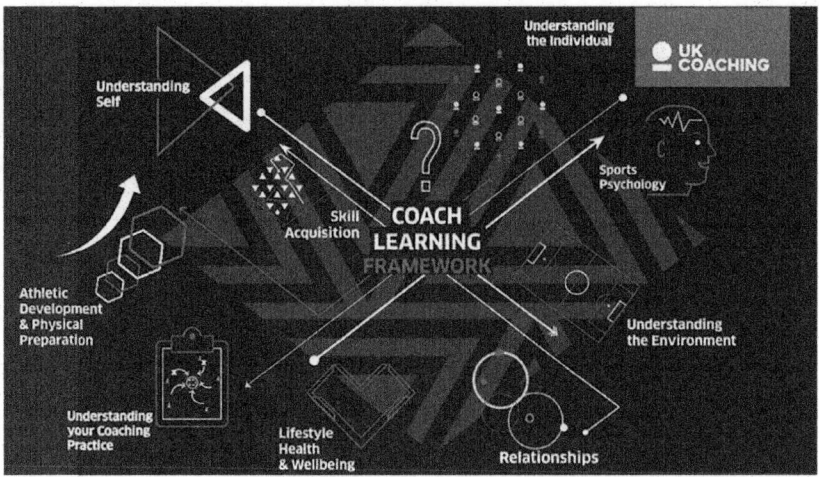

FIGURE 5.1 Coach learning framework. With permission from UK Coaching.

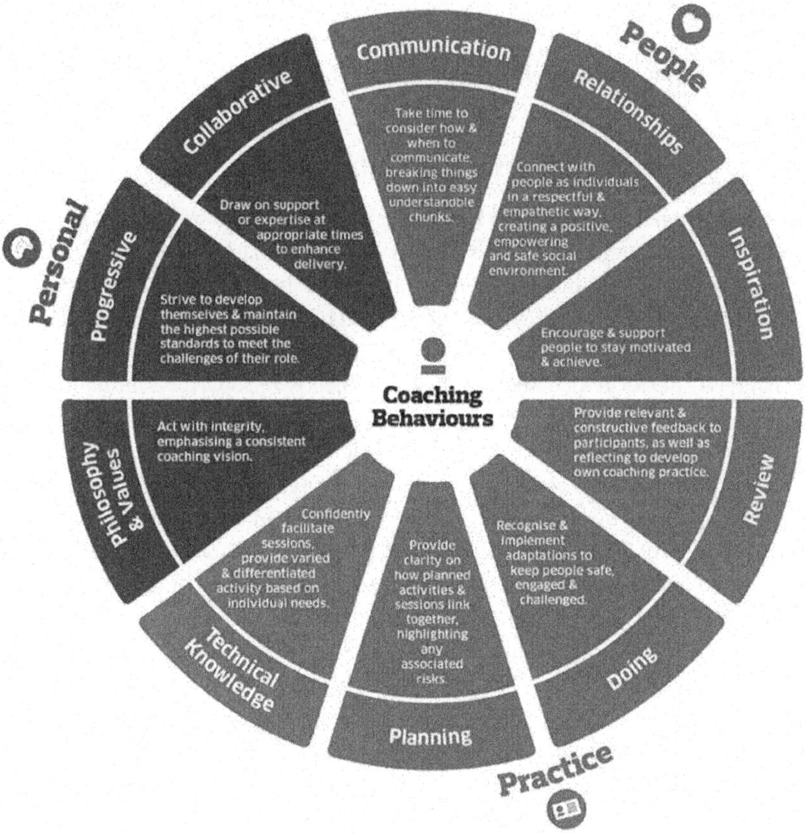

FIGURE 5.2 Coach learning behaviours (sphere). With permission from UK Coaching.

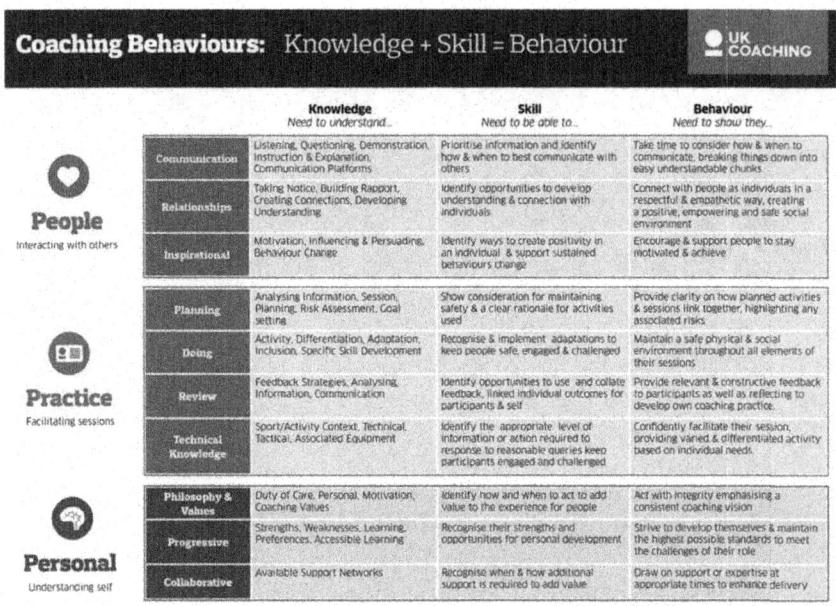

FIGURE 5.3 Coach learning behaviours (matrix). With permission from UK Coaching.

Systematic versus Non-systematic Observation

Everything we have discussed so far is largely based around subjective interpretations of behaviours and opinion-led reflection by the coach. As outlined in Chapter 1 of this book, the human memory has recall limits, and it is reported that coaches memory of critical events within matches and training is relatively low. This presents an information deficit which must be filled, and as per our writing in Chapter 1, performance analysis with its objective properties can help fill this void in regard to remembering and acting upon technical and tactical information. It also means there is an information deficit for the coach when reflecting on their own practice and behaviours when delivering. Some coaches might opt to undertake a form of non-systematic observation of themselves coaching, attempting to get recorded video and then using generic software, observation sheets, self-imposed checklist criteria or similar to generate some form of data. But these are all untried and untested. Given that the coach is likely to be coming up with these tools themselves they will be filled with personal bias and preference about what to look for. Reliability issues will be present too since it is likely that the coach themselves will be the one undertaking the notation, whilst there will be little to no check around validity either. Resultantly this means that without some form of help, the reflection that the coaches are undertaking is unreliable.

To provide a more accurate and astute reflection on coaching delivery, there is a need for a sound conceptual framework to guide the coach. Systematic observation involves a trained observer using a pre-set guideline to observe, record and analyse behaviours. Used in multiple fields not limited to coaching, systematic observation focusses on the use of a pre-set criteria to record actions and behaviours of a professional of interest (e.g. the coach) in relation to the environment and other external influencing factors (Garcia-Lopez, 1988). The method offers the opportunity to produce valid and reliable data about the coach which can be relied upon as an effective manner by which to analyse behaviours.

Coach Analysis Tools

In order to help analyse the behaviours and performance of coaches in a systematic and objective manner, there are a number of tools developed specifically for this purpose, and a growing body of empirical research evidence utilising them. Each holds objective properties which allow coaches to gain a structured insight into the behaviours that they are exhibiting and the frequency at which they use each. Some of these have been utilised alongside performance analysis technologies, though the prevalence of this varies, as discussed below.

Arizona State University Observation Instrument

The Arizona State University Observation Instrument (ASUOI) is a systematic observation instrument consisting of 14 behaviours as displayed in Table 5.1 (Lacy and Darst, 1984). Initially, the traits would be observed and collated on a simplistic notational tally sheet, broken down in relevant sections (such as time divided blocks or elements of the session or game). Each instance would be recorded as a 'mark', with little or no context. Whilst providing a quantified approach of identified behaviours and offering an analysis of sorts, it lacks wider impact. Also, as it is often completed as a live task or observation, the actual recall of events may be lacking, unless accompanied by a recording of the session. The behaviours used in this system have been used in the past for some empirical research studies, and some attempts have also been made to turn the system into an analysis enabled tool, via creating a manual code window in an analysis software.

UK Coaching Observation Checklist

UK Coaching, as part of the 'Analysing your Coaching' workshop, proposed a number of coach behaviours for observation via their observation checklist, split into key sections such as pre-delivery planning, safety, personal qualities and general coaching approach. Other areas included those related to communication, observation and feedback which are critical to the effective delivery of coaching to end users (Figure 5.4). Although a useful guide and including some relevant behaviours, given that each are marked via an 'outcome' this lends itself to subjective interpretation and bias, akin to the properties of non-systematic observation which we earlier critiqued.

TABLE 5.1 Arizona State University observation instrument

	Behaviour	Definition
1	Use of first name	Using the first name or nickname when speaking directly to a player
2	Pre-instruction	Initial Information given to player(s) preceding the desired action to be executed
3	Concurrent instruction	Cues or reminders given during the execution of the skill or play
4	Post-instruction	Correction, re-explanation or instructional feedback given after the execution of the skill or play
5	Questioning	Any question to player(s) concerning strategies, techniques, assignments, etc. associated with the sport
6	Physical assistance	Physically moving the players body to the proper position or through the correct range of motion of a skill
7	Positive modelling	A demonstration of correct performance of a skill or playing technique
8	Negative modelling	A demonstration of incorrect performance of a skill or playing technique
9	Hustle	Verbal Statements intended to intensify the efforts of the player(s)
10	Praise	Verbal or non-verbal compliments, statements or signs of acceptance
11	Scold	Verbal or non-verbal behaviours of displeasure
12	Management	Verbal statements related to the organisational details of a practice session not referring to strategies or fundamentals of the sport
13	Un-codable	Any behaviour that cannot be seen or heard or does not fit into the above categories
14	Silence	Periods of time when the participant is not talking

Coach Analysis Intervention System

Developed by Professor Chris Cushion at Loughborough University, Coach Analysis Intervention System (CAIS) is a multi-dimensional computerised coach behaviour observation system that has identified a combination of 23 primary coaching behaviours and a number of secondary behaviours (Cushion et al., 2012). Primary behaviours relate to physical behaviour, feedback/reinforcement, instruction, verbal/non-verbal language, questioning and session/athlete management. Meanwhile, secondary behaviours relate largely to the contextual additions such as timing, recipients, content, questioning type, silence and practice type in addition to an 'other/transition' category. CAIS uses an online system of specific templates built for these behaviours, focussing on each of the behaviours with their associated secondary counterparts. A trained observer will code each as the session is delivered by the coach, in order to (if deemed suitable) provide live instant feedback. Post-session, the behaviours coded can be synchronised to recorded video before analysis can begin.

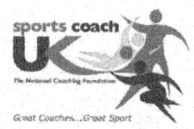

sports coach UK Developing Your Coaching – Analysing Your Coaching

Handout 1 – Prompt Observation Checklist

Did the coach do or consider the following?	Outcome	Comments
Pre-delivery Planning **Did the session plan:**		
have objectives and goals linked to the stage of development/national curriculum if required		
show logical progression		
identify adequate resources and time needed		
have adaptations and alternatives		
show coaching tips and points.		
Safety		
Check the environment and ensure it was safe at all times		
Maintain control of the group and ensure safety at all times		
Maintain control of equipment and ensure safety at all times		
Check participants introduced themselves and the session		
Personal Qualities and General Coaching Approach		
Talk to participants before the session and outline session goals		
Create a 'feel good' factor for all		
Provide variety and challenge		
Maximise involvement		
Have the ability to motivate and inspire		
Stay composed, even under pressure		
Take initiative to make things happen for the better		
Cater for all abilities		
Organisation and Management		
Manage participants effectively		
Manage equipment effectively		
Manage time effectively		
Manage space effectively		
Manage conflict effectively		
Group participants appropriately		

sports coach UK Developing Your Coaching   Analysing Your Coaching

FIGURE 5.4   UK Coaching observation checklist.

Source: With permission from UK Coaching.

Instruction		
Explain the task and skill		
Identify key coaching points		
Develop the session in a progressive way		
Use clear and accurate demonstrations		
Communication Skills		
Gain attention before giving info/demo		
Continually check for understanding		
Ensure adequate voice projection, clarity		
Ensure effective positioning and body language, including maintaining eye contact		
Observation and Feedback		
Have an awareness of the whole group while dealing with individuals		
Provide constructive feedback to participants on performance		
Ask for feedback		
Have an ability to manage success and failure.		

FIGURE 5.4 (Continued).

CAIS is now perhaps the leading tool in this area of coach learning and development. To that end, there has been a plethora of research invested in the use of the tool for helping aid coach development. Various studies have considered the relevant use of the tool in practice towards aiding alterations to coach behaviour to great effect including Harvey et al. (2013) who discovered some changes to coach behaviour after use of the tool. Elsewhere, Hall et al. (2022) investigated the relationship between coach ideology and coaching philosophy, whilst Raya-Castellano et al. (2020) investigated coach behaviour in video feedback sessions, in a direct correlating link to our discipline of performance analysis.

Performance Analysis and Coach Development

Given its objective properties and cemented stature as a sports science discipline, it should not be surprising that the area and influence of performance analysis has emerged to play a significant role in informing the coach and helping them to manage the coaching process (Francis & Jones, 2014). As a form of systematic observation, our discipline offers up the opportunity to enable coaches to reflect with more objectivity and fact and to enhance their reflective processes by providing information to help critically challenge. Wright et al. (2013) state the relevant observation and the ability to assess performance are considered the primary roles of a coach and it should be considered to be crucially important within any level, environment and context of sport and performance for the coach to have the ability to evaluate their own athletes' performances and provide feedback appropriate corrective feedback (Nelson & Groom, 2012; Fernandez–Echeverria et al., 2019). This is key area of influence that the more sustained and relevant use of performance analysis can be developed further as a support mechanism within the coaching process, as it allows for an objective interpretation of the complex reality of performance and the environment in which performance improvement occurs (Butterworth et al., 2013; Fernandez-Echeverria et al., 2019). It is worth noting here that performance can be from an athlete perspective, but in our use of the term here, also the performance of the coach.

This is ultimately where the performance analyst can support the coach in their development, by understanding the coaching process and being able to objectively analyse the coaches coaching performance. By observing the key areas of action and the coach's own behavioural traits, performance analysis can play a significant role in helping enable forward thinking, objective and reliable reflective processes for coaches. This means that the analyst is using their skill set in a different way, transferring the objective and systematic nature of their technical and tactical analysis to the coach, using many of the tools, technologies and processes that they do in their everyday roles. The importance of this role cannot be understated and is becoming increasingly popular as a means by which to gain performance enhancements, after all, if we can help increase the effectiveness of the coaching delivery, we are ultimately still helping increase the overall performance of our athletes.

Using performance analysis in this way is an exciting and developing area, whereby an analyst can craft and apply their skills in an alternative way. For some, the role is becoming embedded within their daily duties, working closely with the coach, coach developer or other senior figures to deliver insights into coach behaviours. For others, entire roles are now dedicated to this, with Aston Villa FC and Glasgow Rangers FC both organisations who have full-time performance analysts dedicated to coach behaviour analysis. The role uses many of the same skills as a 'normal' analyst and is embedded with the same working processes, just working with a different set of data. For those breaking into the industry, knowing, engaging and working with this type of analysis workflow might be one of the things that helps you to 'stand out' in our popular and often oversubscribed employment market.

The Performance Analyst as a Coach Developer

Sport Australia defines the role of a coach developer as to provide ongoing support, advice and encouragement to the coach, with a core focus towards hands-on helping the coach (Sport Australia, 2022). This definition lends itself towards viewing the performance analyst as a coach developer of sorts, assisting via the capture and collection of behavioural data using one of the systematic observation tools we earlier discussed. Of course, there are many other coach developers too including those in that role by title, those in mentoring capacities, other coaches or perhaps even players, all of whom might act as a critical friend in reviewing and deliberating the objective behavioural analysis that is produced.

So as a performance analyst, if you are to become directly involved in the analysis of coach behaviour, it is vital that you able to identify and understand the key traits and behaviours that a coach will exhibit. An initial step towards this is becoming familiar with the behaviours listed in the tools available, be that ASUOI or CAIS, to ensure full appreciation of the behaviours and an ability to observe them in practice. In addition, you might take time considering the context and timing of the session, the environment and level and the perceived outcomes (perhaps via the session plan or wider planned goals through periodic or seasonal plans), so that you can begin to assess if the aims have been met via the behaviours displayed.

Camera, Sounds and Action: Practical and Technological Considerations

Undertaking coach behaviour analysis takes considerable thought and deliberation. To help with this process, Figure 5.5, a model of undertaking coach behaviour analysis has been produced, acting as a practical guide from start to finish, with the following descriptions in text helping analysts to understand the practicalities behind the process.

Marked with a star, the starting place before any behaviour coding or filming takes place, is the analyst carefully understanding the contextual requirements of the coach. Agreeing the focus of the analysis to be undertaken is critical, with all parties clear about the question being set and intended outcomes, which will likely need to be considered together in meetings and potentially ongoing as part of a longer term, wide ranging developmental process. Opening behaviours up to be scrutinised takes a level of humility on behalf of the coach and so it is vital that the relationship gets off to the best possible start with a shared ethos of learning and development being at the centre of the work being undertaken. For the coach, this work will be linked to their own philosophy and reflective cycles, being enhanced with objective data. It is vital then that the analyst is aware of these in situ so that they can help contribute towards this and be aware of the intended outcomes. Indicator development will be considered via selection of an appropriate technological tool and which raw data variable behaviours to code, which will also need to be an agreed decision as all parties look to settle upon

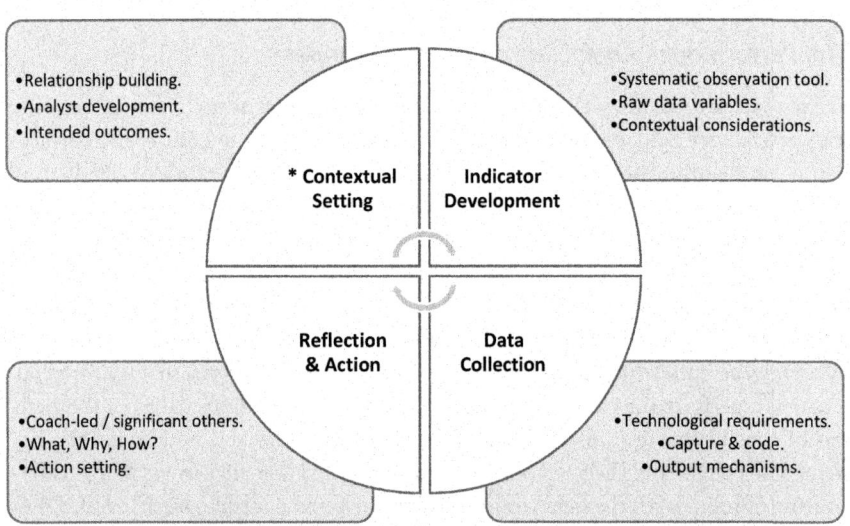

FIGURE 5.5 Coach behaviour analysis cycle.

what will be coded and in what format. For this perhaps utilising some of the existing tools, backed by empirical research will be a sound choice, considering specific contextual nuances in the environment.

As with analysing training and matches, we must carefully consider data collection. In this case, where we seek to code behaviours, that comes as video and data of the coach delivering so that we can *see* what the coach is doing and *hear* what the coach is saying. To capture those data streams effectively, analysts will need to carefully consider the technologies required to do this. A multi camera approach is of huge benefit, given that different perspectives of the same session offers opportunity for a more reliable analysis of behaviours and responses. A three-camera set up would be ideal for this, with a 'wide-angle' sessional view, a coach focused 'tight' view and a body cam 'up-close' view from the coach's perspective. The combination of multiple angles offers an all-round perspective, much as the same way in which analysts seek to take in multiple angles of play from matches. The interpretation of occurrences differs depending on the angle viewed from, for example, the interpretation of players movements, decisions and actions from a position behind the goal compared to a position to the side of the pitch can be very different, much like the interpretation of coach behaviours will differ significantly from a wide angle to an up-close bodycam perspective. A reliable audio feed would also underpin the observations, and the analysis of interpretation of tone of voice along with body language. The addition of an audio feed for the observer may also be highly relevant in some cases, as the analyst may sit a distance away from the coach delivering and so require the audio in order to accurately code the behaviours.

Analysts need to consider if they are seeking to capture and code the coach behaviours live or post-event, in line with requirements from the coach themselves, the coach developer (if in place) and the relevant technology being available. If the work is to take place live, there is a significant investment needed on behalf of the analyst to upskill to the point where they can accurately code in the moment, keeping up with the number of behaviours taking place in situ. This may include completing practice codes and reliability checking with another trained operator on previously captured footage, or may come in the form of practice live codes too on the same (or another) coach to ensure coding can be completed accurately.

The analyst will also need to consider the code window and output mechanisms of the coach behaviours too. A bespoke code window will need to be created which contains the behaviours, and options to add in additional notes for the contextual and environmental factors as required. This will no doubt take some time and should be invested in wisely, alongside the coach themselves and again the coach developer or mentor. An output window which can display the behaviours may also be considered, designing this in an innovative and creative manner which effectively lands the message with the end user, in our case, the coach. This is especially critical if the coach is seeking to have real-time insights into their behaviours, displaying them in a clear and logical manner perhaps with the aid of graphics and imagery built into the software of choice. The analyst must also consider the technological practicalities, deliberating the positioning of cameras, wiring, networking and other infrastructure needs, all of which are discussed elsewhere in this book.

Once the data files have been produced, an analysis of the behaviours can begin and outcomes considered. The purpose of our chapter at this point is not to critically consider the exact methodologies by which that happens, as it is expected that analysts will find value in following the guidelines and recommendations made in the excellent coach behaviour analysis literature body for that purpose. Instead here, we consider *who* might be undertaking this analysis with the coach, *what* they might be reflecting on, and the role that analysts might play. Our model suggests that the coach might consider undertaking the analysis of data themselves, part of their own reflective cycle which we earlier considered. However, the chief problem there is that the coach may interpret and analyse the data in the way that they want to see it, with a lens as to the real meaning that sits behind the data. This may result in no tangible change being made if the coach is not fully honest with themselves, nor able to consider the true meaning of the data set presented to them. Therefore, they might benefit from taking in conversations with significant others, perhaps another coach who can check and challenge the meaning of the data, or a coach developer, mentor or other senior figure. If they're feeling really brave, maybe even the players, who are perhaps likely to be the most honest. Lastly, and most pertinent to the analysis community, the coach might consider being in conversation with ourselves (Figure 5.6), or perhaps ourselves and another coach too.

After all, our discipline promotes objectivity and facts, being able to correlate data points together and consider appropriate next steps. That mirrors well in what the coach is trying to achieve when undertaking a form of analysis on their own behaviours. For us, as performance analysts, this again highlights the importance of analysts knowing coaching. If we do invest time in learning about the discipline more, we can then deepen our understanding of the conceptual process in which we work and be a meaningful part of the critical coach conversations. And so, in being part of this process for the analyst, they'll also be developing at the same time, learning a new way in which to apply their analytical skills whilst also learning more about the coaching environment and process

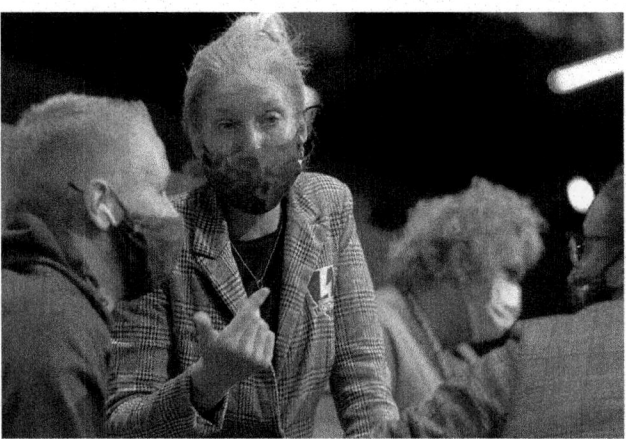

FIGURE 5.6 Coach/analyst conversation.

within which they work. We do though have to know our place, and the coach may not want us to be involved in the analysis of the behaviours, instead only helping to provide the video, audio and coding to support.

As for what the coach will be reflecting upon, it will be explicitly linked to the initial outcomes that were set during stage one of this process. After all, every piece of analysis should have a set question being investigated. The coach may elect to reflect on the behaviours seen in respect of their coaching philosophy and delivery pedagogy, seeking to understand if the alignment is on track with expectations and aims. The contextual environment plays a pivotal part in many coaching scenarios and so this too may be important, alongside assessing behaviours against intended and actual session outcomes. Indeed, from the coach's perspective, they should be able to identify *what* they are coaching and reflect upon its success compared to intended outcomes, using the available data to identify the behaviours they utilise in doing so. There should also then be a consideration of *why* they are coaching what they are coaching, contextualising this conversation back to the environment and other impacting factors. An advantage of involving a performance analyst within these conversations might be that whilst they are observing and coding coaching behaviour, they will also be aware of the reasons and influences on the coaching sessions themselves and the impact on performance data, so can subsequently contribute in a holistic conversation. All of this helps the coach to understand *how* they are coaching, and critically consider actions they need to implement to enhance their practice and delivery back within the coaching process.

Further Considerations for Use

In undertaking analysis of coach behaviours those involved will also need to critically consider how often the work is undertaken. For those with full-time coach analysts, this may become common place or even mandatory, linked to job development reviews. A consideration too is needed around when the analysis is undertaken, which sessions it is done within and the contextual changes that might bring. Analysing a coach in a training environment may bring different views to an analysis undertaken in a match scenario. The analyst's workload too must be considered, since this is a time intensive task with significant manual coding.

The prevalence and use of performance analysis as a coach development tool is not yet widespread. Many coaches reflect on their delivery, but few do it with the objective aid of analysis as described here. This is perhaps not surprising though since within formal coach education courses, performance analysis barely gets a fleeting mention for most. Formal education courses in badminton, football, rugby and cricket make little to no mention of including content around using performance analysis as an objective aid to coach education and development. Some do make mention of the use of analysis in traditional technical and tactical analysis to aid performance reviews, but the innovative use of analysis as a coach development tool with objectively informed coding and analysis is not yet transcending. And so though these courses are for some the start of formal education, the majority do not include performance analysis and so they do not provide the opportunity for a foundational base to introduce and further underpin their perceptions of coaching, as well as challenging convention. Very few coaches link their valued learning to such courses (Jones & Wallace, 2005), as Mallet et al. (2009) considered, most coaches view formal qualifications having little impact in developing their coaching knowledge. However, Lyle (2007) has often stated that coach education should be the key driver for raising coaching standards. Perhaps then there is a need for a wider rethink of coach education courses, inclusive of innovative and effective mechanisms for educating and supporting coaches.

Concluding Remarks

Inherently messy and hard to manage, coaching is a profession traditionally filled with subjectivity and bias. In contrast, performance analysis is a discipline enveloped in fact, objectivity and evidence. Combining the two together provides coaches a meaningful, structured and systematic manner in which to reflect upon their practice and make meaningful changes to behaviours. This presents a rare controllable in the usually messy coaching process, with this facet providing something over which the coach has total control. Bringing the objective properties of analysis into this domain provides many benefits for the coach linked to their professional development and extricable to their philosophical and pedagogical approaches to coaching delivery. Analysis benefits too, with analysts learning more about the environment in which they operate, and helping to provide another objective aid to the exciting and ongoing development of sporting excellence.

References

Abraham, A., Collins, D., Morgan, G., & Muir, B. (2009). *Developing expert coaches requires expert coach development: Replacing serendipity with orchestration.* Leeds Beckett.

Burton, D., & Raedeke, T.D. (2008). *Sport psychology for coaches.* Human Kinetics.

Butterworth, A., O'Donoghue, P., & Cropley, B. (2013). Performance profiling in sports coaching: A review. *International Journal of Performance Analysis in Sport, 13*(3), 572–593.

Cote, J., & Gilbert, W. (2009). An integrative definition of coaching effectiveness and expertise. *International Journal of Sports Science and Coaching, 4*(3), 307–323.

Cross, N. (1995). Coaching effectiveness in hockey: A Scottish perspective. *Scottish Journal of Physical Education, 23*(1), 27–39.

Cushion, C.J., Armour, K.M., & Jones, R.L. (2003) Coach education and continuing professional development: Experience and Learning to Coach. *Quest, 46,* 153–163.

Cushion, C., Harvey, S., Muir, B., & Nelson, L. (2012). Developing the coach analysis and intervention system (CAIS): Establishing validity and reliability of a computerised systematic observation instrument. *Journal of Sports Sciences, 30*(2), 201–216.

Fernandez-Echeverria, C., Mesquita, I., Conjero, M., & Perla Moreno, M. (2019). Perceptions of elite volleyball players on the importance of match analysis during the training process. *International Journal of Performance Analysis in Sport, 19*(1), 49–64.

Francis, J., & Jones, G. (2014). Elite Rugby union players perceptions of performance analysis. *International Journal of Performance Analysis in Sport, 14*(1), 188–207.

Garcia-Lopez, M.D. (1988). Systematic observation of behaviours and environmental events using the lag method. *Perceptual and Motor Skills, 67*(1), 255–262.

Gilbert, W.D., & Trudel, P. (2001). Learning to coach through experience: Reflection in model youth sport coaches. *Journal of teaching in physical education, 21*(1), 16–34.

Hall, J., Cope, E., Townsend, R.C., & Nicholls, A.R. (2022). Investigating the alignment between coaches' ideological beliefs and academy philosophy in professional youth football. *Sport, Education & Society, 27*(3), 377–392.

Harvey, S., Cushion, C., Cope, E., & Muir, B. (2013). A season long investigation into coaching behaviours as a function of practice state: The case of three collegiate coaches. *Sports Coaching Review, 2*(1), 13–32.

Jones, R.L. Armour, K.M., & Potrac, P. (2004). *The cultures of coaching.* London: Longman.

Jones, R., & Kingston, K. (2013). *An introduction to sports coaching: Connecting theory to practice.* London: Routledge.

Jones, R.L., & Wallace, M. (2005). Another bad day at the training ground: Coping with ambiguity in the coaching context. *Sport Education and Society, 10*(1), 119–134.

Klein, G. (2010). *Seeing what others don't—The remarkable way we gain insights.* London: Nicholas Brearley Publishing.

Kolb, D., & David, A. (2014). *Experimental learning: Experience as the source of learning and development.* FT Press.

Lacy, A.C., and Darst, P.W. (1984). Evolution of a systematic observation instrument: The ASU observation instrument. *Journal of Teaching in Physical Education, 3,* 59–66.

Lyle, J. (2002). *Sports coaching concepts.* London: Routledge.

Lyle, J. (2007). Modelling the complexity of the coaching process: A commentary. *International Journal of Sports Science and Coaching, 2*(4), 407–409.

Lyle, J., & Cushion, C. (2017). *Sports coaching concepts: A framework for coaching practice.* Abingdon, UK: Routledge.

Mallet, C., Trudel, P., Lyle, J., & Rynne, S. (2009). Formal vs informal coach education. *International Journal of Sports Science & Coaching, 4*(3), 325–334.

Nelson, L., & Groom, R. (2012). The analysis of athletic performance: Some practical and philosophical considerations. *Sport, Education and Society, 17*(5), 687–670.

Raya-Castellano, P.E., Reeves, M.J., Littlewood, M., & McRobert, A.P. (2020). An exploratory investigation of junior-elite football coaches' behaviours during video-based feedback sessions. *International Journal of Performance Analysis in Sport, 20*(4), 729–746.

Saury, J., & Durand, M. (1998). Practical knowledge in expert coaches: On-site study of coaching in sailing. *Research Quarterly for Exercise and Sport, 69,* 254–266.

Schön, D. (1983). *The reflective practitioner: How professionals think in action.* New York: Basic Books.

Sport Australia (2022). *What is a coach developer and what do they do?* Retrieved 11th August 2022 from: https://www.sportaus.gov.au/__data/assets/pdf_file/0004/684976/What_is_a_Coach_Developer_and_what_do_they_do.pdf

UK Coaching (2022). *Coaching behaviours.* Retrieved 1st July 2022 from: https://www.ukcoaching.org/resources/topics/guides/coaching-behaviours

Walsh, B. (2009). *The score takes care of itself: My philosophy of leadership.* New York: The Penguin Group.

Watkins, C., & Mortimer, P. (1999). Pedagogy: What do we know? In P. Mortimer (Ed.), *Understanding pedagogy and its impact on learning* (pp. 1–19). London: Paul Chapman.

Wright, C., Atkins, S., Jones, B., & Todd, J. (2013). The role of performance analysts within the coaching process: Performance Analysts Survey 'The role of performance analysts in elite football club settings.' *International Journal of Performance Analysis in Sport, 13*(1), 240–261.

6

MICROPOLITICS AND WORKING AS A PERFORMANCE ANALYST IN SPORT

Luke Gibson and Andrew Butterworth

Introduction

Working in sport can be a messy reality, with numerous people, opinions, attitudes and personalities all contributing to a mixing pot of micropolitics, that is, the various day-to-day social realities that staff have to work in and navigate. Being able to navigate through this is tricky, and known as a micropolitical literacy. Recent empirical studies have begun to illuminate some of the micropolitical realities of working life within professional sport, with such realities resulting from an evolving body of literature that has altered our perception of the nature of the practitioner environment (Huggan et al., 2015; Thompson et al., 2015; Gibson & Groom, 2018, 2019, 2020, 2021). Indeed, such investigations have focussed on the working lives of coaches, fitness coaches and performance analysts, evidencing the micro-political challenges faced by practitioners in negotiating the day-to-day environment of professional sport.

The purpose of this chapter is to introduce the background to, and theoretical concepts of, micropolitics, along with some of the key findings from related literature. We will also provide a discussion that emphasises performance analysts' understanding of the complex and ambiguous nature of professional working life, and some suggestions for improving your ability to navigate the micropolitical terrain.

Background to Micropolitics

Working organisations have been identified as political systems of a kind, with complexities involved in organisational life and constant paradoxes or double blinds (Burns, 1961; Butcher & Clarke, 2003). Leftwich (2005) outlines key elements that make up the political nature of human behaviours as people, resources

DOI: 10.4324/9781003226659-6

and power. Indeed, *people* tend to have conflicting ideas, preferences and interests, governed by *power* and the ability to achieve one's desired outcome and the *resources* available to everyone such as material (land, equipment or money) or non-material (time, status, support and opportunity) in nature. In performance analysis this is no different, with different analysts *(people)*, having conflicting ideas about how the analysis workflows should be undertaken dictated by their position *(power)* using a variety of technologies *(resources)* depending on various socio-economic factors. This is just one example, but it is clear that micropolitics is in all aspects of organisational life, including our discipline. Frequently used throughout the literature, Blasé's (1991, p. 11) definition of micropolitics states that

> micro-politics refers to the use of formal and informal power by individuals and groups to achieve their goals. In large part, political actions result from perceived differences between individuals and groups, coupled with a motivation to use power and influence and/or protect.

Taking this approach to studying organisational life allows us to comprehend the inherent political nature that establishes itself within any circumstance that brings two or more people together in any formal, public, or private setting (Leftwich, 2005). As a result, this approach challenges the widespread conception that politics and political activity occurs solely within political institutions and amongst those who are socialised within such institutions. Instead, Leftwich argues that political activity is a characteristic of everyday social life and that politics is not "simply an unnecessary, temporary" or, a "distasteful phenomenon that we could do without" (p. 107). In fact, politics is vital to our social existence, characterised by intrinsic, necessary and functional features of our everyday lives and working practice. Additionally, Ball (1987) indicates that denying the existence and relevance of micropolitics in effect condemns organisational research as ineffectual, and far removed from the realities of working life in organisations.

The exploration of micropolitics within organisational life has been evident within numerous organisational settings such as schools (e.g. Ball, 1987; Kelchtermans, 2002) and business environments (e.g. Dörrenbächer & Geppert, 2006). Although the use of micro-political theory as a lens to understand the business environment has received significant attention, Potrac and Jones (2009a) have called for similar such theory aimed at understanding the working environment of those in professional sport, and in particular professional football in an attempt to shed light on the 'dark side' of organisational life (Hoyle, 1982). Though this call and much of the research is directly towards football, the findings are relevant across sports and not contextualised solely to a single sport, instead they remain relevant to those working in other sports too.

We have already discussed coaching in the opening chapter of this book, and have come to understand it as a complex and messy process. Building further on the rationalistic illustrations of the practice of coaches (Cassidy et al.,

2004; Jones & Wallace, 2005) additional research has positioned coaching as a power-ridden, everyday pursuit which requires practitioners to manage micro-relations with other stakeholders (e.g. athletes, other coaches, manages, owners) as a principal component of their duties (Potrac & Jones, 2009a). Indeed, research investigating the work of coaches (Potrac & Jones, 2009b; Thompson et al., 2015) suggests that 'face-work' (Goffman, 1959) is not only utilised by coaches working at the elite level of football but also fitness coaches/sport scientists employed within this industry. 'Face' is described as an individual's public self-image which develops with and alongside social interaction, and such 'face-work' is efforts made to maintain that image, with conscious efforts often employed by individuals to achieve 'buy-in' from players that they are responsible for.

Key Theoretical Concepts

Much of the micropolitical theory is drawn from the work of Ball (1987) and Kelchtermans (1993, 1996, 2005, 2009), with Kelchtermans and Ballet (2002) furthering the theoretical framework of micropolitics in understanding working life in school environments and how teachers make sense of their working lives. Key to Kelchtermans' (1993) micro-political inquiry are two frameworks: (1) *subjective educational theory*, which is the personal system of knowledge and beliefs about professional sport that practitioners use to perform their jobs (i.e. 'know how'), and (2) the *personal interpretive framework*, which is the set of beliefs and representations developed over time that operates as a lens through which practitioners perceive their job situation and their behaviours.

Professional Self-Understanding

The *personal interpretive framework* is formed through the career experiences of workers and provides them with a perceived identity of themselves within the workplace, alongside a system of knowledge and beliefs related to their professional activity (Kelchtermans, 1993, 2005; Potrac & Jones, 2009a, 2009b). Here, identity is developed over time and relates to the understanding a practitioner has of themselves and influences the sense-making processes of practitioners in any given situation. While our life experiences reflect who we are, this sense of identity is also developed through reflection on *past* and *future* understandings of the *self*. Kelchtermans' (1993, 2005) notion of the *professional self* is the product of interaction with our environment and consists of five sub-constructs: *self-image*, *self-esteem, job motivation, task perception* and *future prospects*.

Kelchtermans (1993, 2005) explains each, beginning with *self-image*, which reflects how practitioners see themselves, how others see them, and how they would typify themselves as an employee. Practitioners tend to reveal self-image in self-descriptive statements, for example, how they would describe themselves to others. This description is often informed by principles that inform a practitioner's professional behaviour and is aligned with the perceptions of significant others. An example might be an analyst describing themselves as an 'innovative and creative analyst with a skill for effective feedback delivery'. Secondly, *self-esteem* refers to the evaluation of oneself as an employee (i.e. 'how good am I at my job?'). Such reflections lead to either positive or negative levels of self-esteem. Within the context of sport, a coach's sense of self may be mediated by the views of their athletes, much like an analyst's might be by the coach. Additionally, the positive or negative judgements from others play an important role in constructing levels of self-esteem. An analyst might perceive themselves as 'an integral part of the team', if they receive feedback from coaches that helps affirm that positive view. According to Kelchtermans, *job motivation* is reflected in one's directional effort to select, stay in, or leave an employment position (i.e. 'the drive to be an analyst or coach'). Weakened social status or respect among colleagues can also lead to decreases in the job motivation. Therefore, job motivation is interrelated with an employee's self-esteem. Positive feedback and positive results that can be linked to the success of analysis workflows might enhance this for the performance analyst. *Task perception* is referred to as the way employees define their job (i.e. 'what ought I to be doing?'). Moreover, productive relationships with colleagues (i.e. fellow analysts, fitness coaches and coaches) and being recognised as competent are significant in the evaluation of such an understanding. Positive task perception may also include autonomy and cooperation with colleagues, along with a stable work environment. Finally, Kelchtermans (1993, 2005) identified *future prospects* in understanding the professional self. This may include reflective questions such as (i.e. 'how do I see myself in my role in years to come and how do I feel about that?'). Furthermore, the interrelated nature of self-image, self-esteem, job motivation and task perception influences practitioner's perception of future prospects.

Professional Interests

Extending the micropolitical framework, the concept of *professional interests* was introduced to understand micropolitical action (Kelchtermans, 1993, 2009; Kelchtermans & Ballet, 2002). Professional interests form part of Kelchtermans' (2009) subjective educational theory as the "personal system of knowledge and beliefs" (p. 263) about a practitioner's working environment. This system prompts questions such as 'how should I deal with this particular situation?' and 'why should I do it that way?'. Indeed, addressing the above questions will help the practitioner to understand the micropolitical nature of a given situation. Developing an ability to read, judge and act upon a situation is essential to becoming competent and successful in different circumstances.

Consistent with Blasé (1991), Kelchtermans and Ballet (2002) outlined professional interests as central to micropolitical theory. The first category of professional interests is that of *self-interests*. Kelchtermans and Ballet (2002) note that when self-esteem or task perception is threatened, the protection of self-interests tend to emerge. Specifically, self-interests guard integrity and identity. In elaborating, Kelchtermans and Ballet (2002) identify the importance of seeking self-affirmation, coping with vulnerability and visibility. Additionally, the judgement from others is pertinent in searching for self-affirmation. In instances of vulnerability, practitioners sense threats to their professional recognition and social relationships (Kelchtermans, 1996). Relatedly, Blasé (1988) described the vulnerable and visible nature of professional environments as 'working in a fishbowl', where significant others observe and evaluate day-to-day working practices (p. 135).

Material interests reflect the access to specific materials, funds or infrastructure needed for a practitioner to carry out their role. Within the sport context, this may be access to facilities, software or other equipment key to one's day-to-day practice. *Organisational interests* are concerned with roles, positions, procedures, and formal tasks within the working environment. Here, the retention of a job and the consideration of job offers make up key organisational interests for practitioners. Kelchtermans and Ballet (2002) suggested that increased job uncertainty can lead to threatened self-esteem and professional competencies. *Cultural-ideological interests* revolve around the explicit norms, ideals or values manifested within a working environment and the organisational culture. Specifically, Altrichter and Salzgeber (2000) indicate these interests as the embodiment of the interactions and procedures in defining that culture. Finally, *social-professional interests* reflect the interpersonal relationships among practitioners within the organisation. Kelchtermans and Ballet (2002) recognised the need to allow for interactions that positively or negatively affect working conditions (e.g. a climate of mistrust, conflict, suspicion and gossip). Blasé (1988) also described a continuum of political strategies that are either reactive or proactive in nature. Reactive strategies are utilised to maintain, negotiate, and protect professional self-interests. Proactive strategies are utilised to improve a given situation or working conditions. These micropolitical strategies become evident in a variety of actions and behaviours such as talking, pleading, arguing, gossiping, flattering, being silent, avoiding taking sides, accepting extra duties and using humour (Blasé, 1991). However, simply creating a list which sums up all actions or strategies is not relevant or possible, since almost any action can become micro-politically meaningful in a particular context, requiring a response of sorts which may not have been on the list.

Professional Leadership Identity

Recent focus has also addressed the concept of professional leadership identity and the process of constructing a professional leadership identity as a micro political activity (Brown & Coupland, 2015; Croft et al., 2015; Koveshnikov et al., 2016). Indeed, such attention has shed light on the potential for investigating and understanding the working practices of those employed within professional sport. Giddens (1991) describes self-identity as a person understanding the self by reflexivity. Sveningsson and Alvesson (2003) suggest that identity themes are attended to on numerous levels including organisational, professional, social and individual, with some of these being linked when organisational identities are seen to cross over to, or fuel, individual identities. The notion of identity is viewed as critical for a large number of issues, including meaning and motivation, commitment, loyalty, logics of action and decision-making, stability and change, leadership, group and intergroup relations, and organisational collaborations (Sveningsson & Alvesson, 2003). Therefore, exploring concepts of identity, as above, and identity work, as below, have become key when understanding organisational life.

Sveningsson and Alvesson (2003) define identity work as people engaging in a process of forming, repairing, maintaining, strengthening, or revising the constructions that are productive in contributing to the achievement of desired outcomes in the workplace. More generally, specific events, encounters, transitions and surprises, as well as more constant strains, serve to heighten awareness of the constructed quality of self-identity. Koveshnikov et al. (2016) further outlined the power that emerges through the construction of certain situations and relationships. Significantly, they suggest that identities formed are dynamic and relational, due to the constant need for (re)negotiation and (re)construction through and in interactions among those in the organisation with employees making sense of who they are, before taking up alternative positions which subsequently influence how employees perceive themselves, others, and relationships with others.

Micropolitics in Sport

Potrac and Jones (2009b) explored the micro-political strategies of a coach (Gavin – pseudonym) in persuading the players, assistant coach and chairperson to accept his coaching philosophy and methods. Whilst the findings highlighted the political nature of the coaching environment, most interesting was the micro-political strategy used by Gavin to have an assistant coach removed from the club. Indeed, Gavin's actions to manipulate the situation to expose the coach's limitations to outmanoeuvre the coach highlighted the Machiavellian (e.g. cunning) behaviours inherent within the coaching climate. Building on this work, Potrac et al. (2013) illustrated the uncaring nature of the working relationships between coaches. Findings evidenced the insular thought processes of a performance coach relating to his career goals, as well as efforts to increase social status within the unforgiving nature of the coaching environment. Similarly, Purdy et al. (2013, as cited in Potrac et al., 2013) highlighted the political conflict between organisational administrators and coaches by portraying elements of trust and distrust within the everyday working environment. In addition, within the sport of rowing, Purdy and Jones (2011) explored how athletes resist the authority of coaches and their coaching methods. Specifically, findings highlighted the actions of rowers who opposed perceived poor coaching practices, openly challenged and scolded coaches, and complained to senior administrators that were organisationally above the coaches.

Interestingly, the work of Thompson et al. (2015) examined the experiences of a newly appointed fitness coach [a coach responsible for the physical attributes and readiness to train of players] at an English Premier League football club, focussing on the process of becoming 'accepted' within the professional football club environment and amongst his professional peers. Indeed, the findings outlined the political and contested nature of the participant's experiences of starting employment within a professional football club. Thompson et al. (2015) highlighted the impression management that the participant engaged in when trying to present himself "to his new colleagues" (p. 12) and align himself with the current norms and values of the other first team staff. Such findings highlight the influence of the working environment and the micropolitical actions and behaviours of individuals on self-presentation (Goffman, 1959).

Micropolitics in Performance Analysis

Specifically, in our discipline, Huggan et al. (2015) investigated the organisational life of a performance analyst in a professional football club, revealing the vulnerable nature of working in professional football. Though this is the only explicit study into the area thus far, it provides an important insight into some of the struggles faced by a professional analyst, from which readers will learn. Particularly, data evidenced the struggles of getting professional colleagues to buy into the role and the development of an identity that was coherent with the social make-up of organisational life within professional football. Indeed, such factors were perceived to have a significant impact on the success of the individual's performance. Both papers (Huggan et al., 2015; Thompson et al., 2015) support the notion that micro-political activity not only affects the coaching practice, but the working lives of others employed within professional football clubs. Though this research provides an insight into the exact role of analysis and other disciplines, further work examining the interrelated nature of practitioner working life was needed. Therefore, the more recent work of Gibson and Groom (2018, 2019, 2020, 2021) explored the micropolitical complexities of working life in an academy in a professional football club (Alder FC) during a period of organisational change. Participants in the sample referred to their working relationships with analysts and other support staff as part of this work, providing excellent insights into the realities of current working practice in elite environments, with many examples and situations which will resonate with analysts reading this chapter, or make those seeking to go into the industry aware of what may come their way.

A Case Study of Micropolitics in the Academy of a Professional Football Club

Firstly, the authors focussed on the experiences of an academy coach (Ian) employed at Alder FC through the theoretical lens of *professional self-understanding*. Findings highlighted those fellow coaches, who regularly provide professional support and reflective dialogue, would disassociate themselves from Ian when it appeared that he was under scrutiny from senior management figures. Specifically, Ian reported that, "it was as if to say, 'we're nothing to do with this group, or Ian'". Ian also explained how he made sense of the communication within the club, and the political nature of such messages to help individuals strengthen their position and protect their agenda. Indeed, in engaging in such micropolitical action, coaches and leaders within the academy were perceived to be 'stabbing each other in the back'. Interestingly, Ian revealed that he needed to become more 'politically savvy' to the behaviours of professional colleagues to successfully negotiate the working environment of professional football. These findings are likely to be experienced and replicated in other sports too, not just football.

Furthermore, to understand the experiences of practitioners at different organisational levels of the professional football club, Gibson and Groom (2019) continued to investigate the experiences of a head of Foundation Phase (James) at Alder FC. Indeed, James' primary focus was to maintain his position and stay in his role as Head of Foundation Phase and protect his own *professional self-interests*. This desire drove his motivations and his micropolitical actions and strategies within the workplace. Specifically, James took up opportunities to engage in social activities, such as staff five-a-side football games with senior managerial figures, along with informal conversations with academy coaches, who he was responsible for, to ensure that they remained 'onside'. Interestingly, James was also aware of the need to maintain a *social distance* from staff who were perceived to be unfavourable among senior managerial figures.

The experiences of a newly appointed head of Professional Development Phase (Jack) were also examined. Indeed, Gibson and Groom (2020) highlighted how Jack constructed a *professional leadership identity* to influence other staff, win trust, avoid becoming socially isolated, or to be perceived as weak. Such action was understood to significantly influence the protection of his employment status. Interestingly, findings evidenced sources of self-doubt felt by Jack during instances of vulnerability when trying to address the business remit of developing academy players to be sold for a financial profit. Additionally, the remit that Jack was tasked with also required him to appraise the support staff (i.e. fitness coach, physiotherapist, performance analyst) that he would be working with to achieve his goals. In these instances, Jack engaged in *identity work* to evaluate whether each staff member would support him in being successful in his job role.

Finally, focussing on the experiences of the Academy Manager (Richard) at Alder FC, Gibson and Groom (2021) evidenced the need for Richard to negotiate employment vulnerability, complexity and ambiguity to strategically respond to the actions and behaviours of senior figures such as the first team manager, chairman and board of directors. For example, this included 'selling ideas' to the first team manager, managing perceptions and expectations of the first team manager and politically championing alternative courses of action. In such instances, Richard's socio-cultural understanding of the working context guided his actions and behaviours when it came to deciding on when to 'go up against' the first team manager and when to 'back down'. When backing down, Richard developed an emotional coping strategy to deal with these micropolitical situations. Similarly, Richard was also required to manage those below him. This prompted Richard to deal with situations where some coaches would be resistant to change, whilst engaging in micropolitical activity to win trust and respect with other coaches.

The case study findings highlight the interrelated nature of micropolitics within the academy at a professional football club. That is, all participants with various organisational roles and responsibilities engaged in some form of micro-political activity and highlighted the need to understand the micropolitical essence that can often drive the actions and behaviours of others, particularly during periods of organisational and managerial change. Specifically, the working practices, the working environment and professional working relationships were all characterised as micropolitical in some manner. Indeed, notions of vulnerability were experienced by all four participants within the case study; however, the sources of that vulnerability were influenced by the role of each participant, and where they sat within the organisational hierarchy (i.e. the Academy Manager's professional working relationship with the Chairperson, or the working environment of the Academy Coach).

Interestingly, the case study evidenced the ambiguous nature of working life in a professional football club and how such ambiguity was driven by poor communication from related, senior colleagues. These situations prompted unanswered questions such as, 'what am I doing right/wrong?' and led to participants' negative *professional self-understanding*. Furthermore, findings highlighted that when participants' *professional self-interests* were 'protected', their working environment and working practices became more favourable, leading to a more positive perception of organisational life within their professional football club.

Why Do Performance Analysts Need to Understand Micropolitics?

As highlighted above, working life in professional sport is inherently micropolitical. Indeed, the development of one's micropolitical literacy is a requirement regardless of role, or level in the organisational hierarchy. That is, analysts employed within professional sport may need to navigate the micropolitical context of a variety of situations or events within their working life. For instance, a recently employed analyst in a new club may need to understand the micropolitical context of their new working environment by developing a level of 'social astuteness' through the incisive observation of others (Munyon et al., 2015). In doing so, we may consider the work of Ball (1987) in his attempt to get teachers to understand the micropolitical environment of the school. Adapting Ball's (1987) work within the context of professional sport may prompt analysts to reflect on (a) the key influential actors within their new club, (b) how key decisions are made, (c) the managerial style of the head coach/first team manager/

head of department, (d) who supports and challenges the head coach/first team manager/head of department and (e) the conduct of meetings. In practical terms that might be the analyst taking a 'back seat' in initial weeks, seeking to observe the working practices of various stakeholders in the environment and learning about them. The same might be true of players, where the analyst might seek to understand players by observation and reflection. For both, the analyst might also employ the strategy of 'getting to know' them away from the job role or indeed sport at all, to build a rapport in a tactic to bring them 'onside' early in the analyst's career in the environment.

Following an understanding of these issues, and when presented with related situations, analysts may engage with reflective questions as suggested by Jones et al. (2011). Such questions may consist of "what to say to whom, when and how? What would be the consequences of such actions? And is the social cost worth it?" (p. 3) (i.e. "you can't go to war with the 1st Team Manager, you won't win" [Gibson & Groom, 2019, p. 16]). Answers to such questions will guide behaviour as a practitioner and may be further informed by thinking about their own self-image (i.e. how you would describe yourself to other analysts, coaches, fitness coaches, players etc. at the club) and self-esteem (i.e. how others would describe/judge you in your role as an analyst) (Kelchtermans, 1993). Furthermore, in their exploration of the narrative story of a performance analyst working in professional football, Huggan et al. (2015) found that being perceived as a 'proper' performance analyst and competent in their role as a performance analyst was desirable feature of their professional life. Whilst most accept analysis as a 'proper science' now, there are still some reluctant to accept this, and so there may be scenarios where the analyst feels that they have to justify their role in some way, to become an accepted part of the organisation.

Reflecting on the above issues may also inform how analysts 'sell' ideas to senior figures within the club; a key skill set when 'managing up' within organisational life (Gibson & Groom, 2021). Here, Kelchtermans and Ballet's (2002) framework of *professional interests* becomes apparent when deciding on micropolitical action. For example, a leader may need to carefully consider the best approach to protect their material interests if they require financial support for department resources (i.e. new software and equipment) to enhance practice and productivity within their team. When engaging in such action, one may need to understand "what the powers that be are like, what potentially could they do with this problem... if something needs weight behind it, going to the Chairman or a money man might be the answer" (Gibson & Groom, 2020, p. 773). Analysts might also think tactically about how to explain to and, gain the understanding of the decision makers about the value that a certain new product brings them. Drawing upon some of the content in Chapters 2 and 10 of this book may also provide guidance here. A sound pedagogical approach to investing in analysis infrastructure is critical, as is finding the optimal solution based upon budgetary confines, thus there will be a need to think this through thoroughly before going 'up' to have conversations.

As discussed, leading a department of analysts requires a level of micropolitical skill. Such an endeavour not only requires an individual to manage-up (i.e. head coach/first team manager/sporting director), but to also manage those hierarchically below in your team of analysts. Here, one may consider the social group identity of the team they are responsible for, and how the creation of their own professional leadership identity is aligned to that of the group. As outlined by Gibson and Groom (2020), leaders may be required to consistently revise and maintain their professional leadership identity as the micropolitical landscape evolves, and their micropolitical literacy becomes increasingly informed. Indeed, a new head of performance analysis may have to "fit into them [their team] first, get their trust... rather than isolate" themselves (Gibson & Groom, 2020, p. 772) before implementing desired or required changes to working practices. In doing so, the leader is protecting their own self-interests by getting their staff 'onside' (Gibson & Groom, 2019).

For analysts working early in their careers, the considerations of micropolitical literacy will likely be vast and varied, riddled perhaps with self-doubt or imposter syndrome, especially early on if part of a 'big' organisation which brings its own pressures. Therefore, noting an awareness of your own *professional self* is critical. *Self-image* will likely be a big consideration early in a career, with analysts perhaps cautious of 'overselling' themselves early on in fear of being found out or, the other extreme by over-promoting themselves, only to be found out later on and thus damaging relations. Both of these are of course explicitly linked to *self-esteem* in obvious ways. The notion of *job motivation* is unlikely to be an issue early into an analyst's career, especially if you have landed a dream job. Motivation is therefore going to be present, though that should not stray into over eagerness or knowing place, at which point issues of *task perception* may come into play whereby analysts define their job up or down. For those engaged in and around interns or placements these issues might be further heightened as they seek to do all they can to impress over the duration of their role in order to try and secure a job at the end, which may or may not be in the pipeline. This is a consideration of *future prospects* for analysts, with interrelated issues also attached. A solution would be to engage in reflection through formal means with mentors and significant others to help their own development, requiring a certain level of vulnerability and humbleness, which may harm perceptions. Though the benefits of reflective practice are many, students and early career analysts are notoriously bad at engaging with reflective practice and have pre-conceived poor conceptions of its worth. If, however it is engaged with, the value is huge, helping to navigate some of the many issues we have uncovered in this chapter.

Concluding Thoughts

In summary, we have provided a background to micropolitics, along with some theoretical concepts that have underpinned activity aimed at understanding micropolitics in organisational life and professional sport. Although further exploration of working life in professional sport, and specifically performance analysis, is required, we believe that the need for practitioners to develop their repertoire of micropolitical skill and action is becoming increasingly prevalent. Indeed, good micropolitical literacy may reduce feelings of vulnerability in an environment that is frequently described as unstable, contested, socially complex and fraught with competing agendas amongst stakeholders (Gibson & Groom, 2019). Whilst we cannot provide a definitive, bulletproof guide of behaviours for every micropolitical situation faced as a performance analyst, we believe that reflections on the theoretical concepts and empirical findings discussed in this chapter may better prepare practitioners for considering how their behaviours may influence their day-to-day working life. Moreover, practitioners should dedicate enough of their professional development to understanding the inter-related nature of micropolitical activity and their daily procedural and technical duties within organisational life in professional sport. Indeed, we suggest that in doing so, analysts may become more 'politically savvy' (Gibson & Groom, 2018). Finally, in reflecting on their own experiences, Jones et al. (2011) state, "every utterance seemed to count, every gesture had an effect in terms of se-curing, maintaining, or losing respect of those we wanted to influence" (p.3). Therefore, in your working careers as analysts, carefully consider every action, every thought and every decision, since you may not know the value or harm it may hold.

References

Altrichter, H., & Salzgeber, S. (2000). Some elements of a micro-political theory of school development. In H. Altrichter & J. Elliot (Eds.), *Images of educational change* (pp. 99–110). Buckingham and Philadelphia: Open University Press.

Ball, S. (1987). *The micro-politics of the school: towards a theory of school organization.* London: Methuen.

Blasé, J.J. (1988). The everyday political perspective of teachers: Vulnerability and con-servatism. *International Journal of Qualitative Studies in Education, 1*(2), 125–142.

Blasé, J.J. (1991). *The politics of life in schools.* Newbury Park: Sage.

Brown, A.D., & Coupland, C. (2015). Identity threats, identity work and elite profession-als. *Organization Studies, 36*(10), 1315–1336.

Burns, T. (1961). Micro-politics: mechanisms of institutional change. *Administrative Sci-ence Quarterly, 6*(3), 257–281.

Butcher, D., & Clarke, M. (2003). Redefining managerial work: Smart politics. *Manage-ment Decision, 41*(5), 477–487.

Cassidy, T., Jones, R.L., & Potrac, P. (2004). *Understanding sports coaching: The social, cul-tural and pedagogical foundations of coaching practice.* London: Routledge.

Croft, C., Currie, G., & Lockett, A. (2015). The impact of emotionally important social identities on the construction of a managerial leader identity: A challenge for nurses in the English National Health Service. *Organization Studies, 36*(1), 113–131.

Dörrenbächer, C., & Geppert, M. (2006). Micro-politics and conflicts in multinational corporations: Current debates, re-framing, and contributions of this special issue. *Journal of International Management, 12*, 251–265.

Gibson, L., & Groom, R. (2018). The micro-politics of organisational change in profes-sional youth football: Towards an understanding of 'the professional self.' *Managing Sport & Leisure, 23*(1–2), 106–122.

Gibson, L., & Groom, R. (2019). The micro-politics of organisational change in profes-sional youth football: Towards an understanding of 'actions, strategies and professional interest'. *International Journal of Sports Science & Coaching, 14*(1), 3–14.

Gibson, L., & Groom, R. (2020). Developing a professional leadership identity during organisational change in professional youth sport. *Qualitative Research in Sport, Exercise & Health, 12*(5), 764–790.

Gibson, L., & Groom, R. (2021). Understanding 'vulnerability' and 'political skill' in academy middle management during organisational change in professional youth football. *Journal of Change Management, 21*(3), 358–382.

Giddens, A. (1991). Modernity and self-identity: Self and society in the late modern age. Palo Alto, CA: Stanford University Press.

Goffman, E. (1959). *The presentation of self in everyday life.* New York: Doubleday Anchor Books.

Hoyle, E. (1982). Micro-politics of educational organisations. *Educational Management Administration & Leadership, 10,* 87–98.

Huggan, R., Nelson, L., & Potrac, P. (2015). Developing micro-political literacy in pro-fessional soccer: A performance analyst's tale. *Qualitative Research in Sport Exercise & Health, 7*(4), 504–520.

Jones, R.L., & Wallace, M. (2005). Another bad day at the training ground: coping with ambiguity in the coaching context. *Sport, Education & Society, 10,* 119–134.

Jones, R.L., Potrac, P., Cushion, C., & Ronglan, L.T. (2011). *The sociology of coaching.* London: Routledge.

Kelchtermans, G. (1993). Getting the story, understanding the lives. From career stories to teachers' professional development. *Teaching and Teacher Education, 10,* 443–456.

Kelchtermans, G. (1996). Teacher vulnerability: Understanding its moral and political roots. *Cambridge Journal of Education, 26*(3), 307–323.

Kelchtermans, G. (2005). Teachers' emotions in educational reforms: Self-understanding, vulnerable commitment and micro-political literacy. *Teaching and Teacher Education, 21,* 995–1006.

Kelchtermans, G. (2009). Who I am in how I teach is the message: Self-understnding, vulnerability and reflection. *Teachers and Teaching, 15*(2), 257–272.

Kelchtermans, G., & Ballet, K. (2002). Micro-political literacy: Reconstructing a ne-glected dimension in teacher development. *International Journal of Educational Research, 37,* 755–767.

Koveshnikov, A., Vaara, E., & Ehrnrooth, M. (2016). Stereotype-based managerial iden-tity work in multinational corporations. *Organization Studies, 37*(9), 1353–1379.

Leftwich, A. (2005). The political approach to human behaviour: People, resources and power. In A. Leftwich (Ed.), *What is politics?* (pp. 100–119). Cambridge: Polity Press.

Munyon, T.P., Summers, J.K., Thompson, K.M., & Ferris, G.R. (2015). Political skill and work outcomes: A theoretical extension, meta-analytic investigation, and agenda for the future. *Personnel Psychology, 68*(1), 143–184.

Potrac, P., & Jones, R.L. (2009a). Power, conflict and cooperation: Toward a micro-politics of coaching. *Quest, 61,* 223–236.

Potrac, P., & Jones, R.L. (2009b). Micro-political workings in semi-professional football. *Sociology of Sport Journal, 26,* 557–577.

Potrac, P., Jones, R.L., Gilbourne, D., & Nelson, L. (2013). 'Handshakes, BBQs, and bullets': Shame, self-interest, shame and regret in football coaching. *Sports Coaching Review, 1*(2), 79–92.

Purdy, L., & Jones, R.L. (2011). Choppy waters: elite rowers' perceptions of coaching. *Sociology of Sport Journal, 28*(3), 329––346.

Purdy, L., Potrac, P., & Nelson, L. (2013). Trust, distrust and coaching practice. In P. Potrac, W. Gilbert, & J. Denison (Eds.), *The Routledge handbook of sports coaching* (pp. 309–321). London: Routledge.

Sveningsson, S., & Alvesson, M. (2003). Managing managerial identities: Organizational fragmentation, discourse and identity struggle. *Human Relations, 56*(10), 1163–1193.

Thompson, A., Potrac, P., & Jones, R. (2015). I found out the hard the hard way: Micro-political workings in professional football. *Sport, Education and Society, 20,* 976–994.

7

PERCEPTIONS, VALUE AND EFFICACY OF PERFORMANCE ANALYSIS

Andrew Butterworth

Introduction

Once known as the new kid on the block, performance analysis is no longer regarded as an emerging sports science discipline. Now, it is firmly embedded as an integral part of the coaching process, an important asset for players and coaches alike. Some empirical research suggests that elite football coaches recall just 59% of critical events accurately (Laird & Waters, 2008), and though that number varies in other research it is clear that there are issues with recall and accurate subjective interpretation. This means that there is a significant information deficit, with nearly half of critical events either forgotten or misinterpreted. Further still, the information that is successfully recalled, is likely to be filled with bias, subjectivity and personal prejudice if undertaken without the aid of objectively informed performance analysis. Indeed, research confirms that coach observations are often exaggerated, inaccurate and incomplete (Franks & Miller, 1991).

Performance analysis is largely considered an objective science to help this problem through evidence and fact. Though that said, O'Donoghue (2010) challenges the traditional view of performance analysis as a truly objective science, given that it cannot account for observer bias amongst other issues. However, accepting the view that analysis is more objective and accurate than coach observations alone, we can begin to understand why the prevalence of the discipline has grown. Analysis has become well engrained within the coaching process as it consistently helps plug the information deficit and provide evidence based back up to common performance problems. Recent research confirms the prevalence of use in some settings, reporting that 98% of elite football coaches in England have access to performance analysis (Andersen et al., 2022).

But whilst growth in use is not lacking, what is, is substantiated evidence that it actually works. Given the dynamic and interactive nature of sport, this is

DOI: 10.4324/9781003226659-7

perhaps not surprising, with little in the way of research to show the impacts on performance itself in underlying the undoubted need for analysis provision. With the advent of more closely entwined interdisciplinary practice now becoming more common in elite sport settings, it becomes more difficult still, to prove that it is in fact analysis that makes a difference. It is therefore difficult to gain evidence directly correlating the use of performance analysis to success. Some might question the need to pinpoint the exact means of success at all though, so long as it happens, or indeed if it is ever possible to do so given the dynamic and interactive nature. Regardless of views on that, what is becoming clearer are the various means by which we can attempt to understand and correlate the place, perception and value of our discipline.

Anecdotal evidence reports efficacious use in practice, whilst coaching process models *of* the discipline now chart the role of performance analysis in significant terms. Media coverage, journalistic attention and fan engagement all point towards a growth in acceptance, or at least intrigue. Crossing the academic and practical fields, action research has been undertaken in real empirical settings to try and provide critical insight into the discipline. Action research helps challenge thoughts and pre conceived opinions, whilst gaining important views of key stakeholders. With that contained, it allows for unbiased and critical reflection, seeking to help provide catalytic validity, with the research acting as an agent for change where adjustments are required. Documenting coaches, players and analysts themselves, a body of qualitative work has emerged to try and discover true perceptions and values of performance analysis in practice. It is this work which helps us to better understand and chart the value of analysis, earning insight into details regarding the learning that the role plays.

Perceptions: Coaches

As those ultimately responsible for the success of a team or individual, coaches are the gatekeepers of multiple information sources and are tasked with making decisions either with, or without that information. Guitierrez–Aguilar et al.'s (2016) research evidences the positive role that coaches play in developing better sporting performances, discovering that marked improvements were statistically significant in the periods immediately after reinstruction by coaches. In other words, after coaches intervene and deliver feedback information to their players, it transfers to immediate positive actions on performance. Instances in this research were undertaken and instructions laid without the aid of performance analysis to help. Given the varying suggestions of how much information coaches actually recall from performances, performance analysis has a significant role to play in helping plug that information deficit. To that end, Wright et al. (2012) suggest that performance analysis strongly enhances coaches' feedback during the coaching process, helping to cement the significant importance of the discipline, since with efficacious use in practice to help reinstruction might see further positive actions following feedback, in correlation with findings from

Guitierrez-Aguilar et al.'s (2016) research. Charting the views of coaches on performance analysis is critically important therefore, considering the place of the discipline and the critical role coaches play in connection practitioners and athletes in an ever complicated and messy coaching process.

Empirical models *of* the coaching process situate performance analysis as critical at all stages, providing some documentary evidence that the place of analysis is firmly valued (Mayes et al., 2009; Horne, 2013). These research studies also point to the pivotal consideration of communication, providing empirical suggestions as to the flow and direction of information, to and from athletes, coaches and analysts. These considerations are critical to the effective implementation of analysis workflows if any provisions are to be considered effective and valued. If communication channels are not clear and messages not clearly landed with the end users (e.g. players and coaches), then views and perceptions of analysis may become distorted.

For the majority, where communication is clear and messages do convey to coaches, multiple studies now cite the self-reported value of performance analysis in enhancing decision making, aiding objectivity and clarifying important aspects of play. What is also clear from previous research is that coaches' past experiences and philosophies have a significant impact on their decision making regarding the implementation of performance analysis in practice (Wright et al., 2012; Mooney et al., 2016; Kraak et al., 2018). Considering this, in female sport, Loo et al. (2020) report the positive perception of analysis in Asia in water polo and netball alike. Specifically, the study highlights the important role analysis plays in developing game understanding whilst also providing learning opportunities. Other research into female sports reports similar, with Fernandez-Echeverria et al. (2019) highlighting the value of analysis in a single subject case study of a female volleyball team and De Martin Silva and Francis (2020) citing that over time and with significant use, analysis helps develop tactical knowledge and better results. Empirical research such as this helps us better understand and contextualise the practical worth of the discipline the leads us towards initial important evidence of the role analysis plays in the outcome of match results.

In elite football, early investigations into the discipline emerged, with football coaches queried as to their use areas and recommendations for analysis integration. Groom and Cushion (2004, 2005) elicited positive opinions having undertaken qualitative data collection with elite youth academies, where a number of interesting themes emerged. Support and informing training were highlighted as use areas, whilst motivation, opposition analysis and performance modelling were also cited. The study suggested that a 1:1 ratio of positive feedback was important for performance enhancements with youth athletes and that negative examples should be kept to a minimum for teams or individuals suffering reduced confidence. Perhaps most interesting is the finding that analysis takes away coaches' emotion, allows them to change perspective with a more informed view and to subsequently review matches in a more balanced manner. Directly following on their initial study, Groom et al. (2011) proposed an initial grounded theory for performance analysis which considered delivery approaches and conceptual links to the coaching process.

Wright et al.'s (2012) study provided further weight to the argument that analysis is an effective discipline. In their study of elite coaches, it was suggested that performance analysis is heavily valued and essential to practice, helping to provide the majority of coaches the opportunity to more objectively debrief performances. With regular use, the discipline provides consistency and delivers important insights and data points towards various planning cycles. Interestingly, the work also highlighted the close relationship of coaching philosophy and gut instinct, with nearly all coaches communicating that these inform selection of indicators and of players for matchday squads. This promotes an interesting conversation for the future of performance analysis, wherein the balance of this expert knowledge must be considered in tandem with objective performance analysis, not seen as a rival or challenge.

In other sports, the positive impact analysis has continues to be displayed too. Almeida et al.'s (2019) study with futsal coaches undertook interviews to discover what helps them make decisions. Performance analysis was utilised heavily as a guiding line, with coaches electing to consult the discipline for their own team structure and tactics, before then turning attention to the opposition. There were further clear signs of coaching behaviours that use analysis as cues for decision making and implementation during live competitions, hinting towards the efficacious use of analysis live in the moment. In rugby union, semi-professional South African head coaches confirm that performance analysis supports decision making in their sport too (Kraak et al., 2018).

Spanning multiple sports, it is therefore clear that a sizeable population of coaches help in painting a positive picture of a discipline embedded in subjectivity, evidence and fact, with many concurrent and similar themes regardless of sport or level. Though not all research agrees, with certain demographic groups reported as being less perceptive to use. For example, Butterworth et al. (2012) who discovered older coaches instead largely opt to trust their experience and gut rather than seek objective support through analysis. Martin et al. (2018) suggest potential reasoning for situations such as this, contemplating that those coaches who lack support and education, may subsequently invest less time and therefore lead towards differing or diminished views on the role analysis plays.

Resource also plays a part too, with some stating that they would like to use the discipline more, but are restricted by budgetary constraints. This is true in rugby, with Kraak et al.'s (2018) study uncovering that not all coaches have access and others having to outsource, in Painczyk et al.'s (2017) provincial coach study where only 20% had access and in Danish A-Licence football coaches where only 46% have the access they desire. And so, whilst the integral nature of performance analysis to support coach decision making is rich in evidence, there are remaining barriers to help extend this support across all sports at all levels.

Perceptions: Athletes

The ultimate end users of analysis information are the athletes themselves. It is they who are the ones performing on a match day and so need to be able to take in the information and utilise for the betterment of performance. Their views on the structure, timing and presentation methods by those delivering are therefore imperative to discovering the value efficacious use and worth of analysis. Groom and Cushion (2005) suggest that when planning an analysis approach, it is critical to take into account these athletes' perceptions for practical use. Through both questionnaire and interview data collection, Wright et al.'s (2016) research investigated this through the perceptions of athletes in elite academy and senior football. Athletes responded to confirm that simply having volumes of information is not sufficient, and that players required additional guidance and support to facilitate the identification of cues, alongside supporting *why* conversations for tactical alignment. With help, some athletes were then able to interact and contribute, though some still did not participate with engagement varying considerably. Given the large number of learning differences and contextual factors, this is not surprising, and it remains a difficult role for the coach and analyst to deliver engaging feedback which meets the needs of all their athletes.

Fernandez-Echeverria et al. (2019) further discuss the usefulness of analysis from an athlete perspective, seeking the views of elite volleyball players on the importance of match analysis. The study discovered that athletes' value being able to view their own performances, especially negative aspects, with a developmental view to correction in future games. They also reported positive benefits in regard to opposition analysis, which enabled learning and tactical enhancements before match day. Athletes also reported the motivational benefits of analysis provision, something earlier confirmed in netball research by Jenkins et al. (2007), and the psychological benefits as reported in Reeves and Roberts (2013), both of which help contextualise the multifaceted use of analysis in practice not just for tactical or technical enhancement, but also providing psychological benefits, helping cement the place of analysis firmly within the IDT.

In further understanding the prevalence and use of the discipline for practice, important considerations arise when thinking about the time at which analysis is delivered, with Wright et al.'s (2016) participants suggesting that 24–48 hours should pass before delivery. This is a common view in practice too, with anecdotal evidence from players suggesting that they value the opportunity for emotions to subside before starting to rationally decipher their performances more objectively. Though, recent technological advances have seen the advent of near real-time feedback including the ability to portray data and video in training or match scenarios. Rugby players enjoy the immediate nature of this with Francis and Jones' (2014) participants finding that immediate learning occurs using in the moment video streams, rather than having to wait until after training had passed. Given that 79% of analysts are involved in a form of live analysis, with 43% of coaches utilising this in their decision-making practice, these are important findings for contextualising the worth of analysis by players in practice, adding further value (Wright et al., 2012, 2013).

Further interesting comparisons start to arise when independently considering genders, with Loo et al. (2020) suggesting that there is certain gender-based differences in athlete views and perceptions of analysis, such as motivation and self-led analysis for active tasks, culture and discussions which were positively received with females. This can be directly modelled in comparison to the research of Middlemas and Harwood (2017) whereby coaches significantly invested time in designing similar player-led tasks for males, but engagement and attitudes dropped in the athletes, leading to decreased on pitch performance. Conversely, Wright et al. (2016) earlier stated that male academy players seek to be actively involved in analysis processes, becoming empowered to be a critical part of their own analysis and feedback process. Active athlete involvement does generally appear to be critical to positive engagement, with Moreno-Perla et al. (2016) also highlighting the important role of active learning through questioning, whilst Bampouras et al. (2012) cite athletes' desires to be involved and offer input via questioning. Further support for an active process is contributed by De Martin Silva and Francis (2020), who found over time that increases in tactical understanding, performance outcomes and feelings of belonging were evident, thus providing explicit support for the value and place of analysis by athletes.

Mature views on the financial viability and potential rewards on investment were considered by those taking part in Francis and Jones (2014) study. Rugby players there firstly considered that the club must accept the cost implications of a performance analysis workflow, before then deliberating the usability and uptake of the system. Combined, it is suggested that the outcomes of these views help decipher if it is a wise investment and sensible financial investment. Ice hockey players meanwhile discussed their respect for the discipline, and the coaches who invested considerable time into developing slick presentations, linked to wider tactical outcomes (Nelson et al., 2014). They further suggested that analysts, especially those early in their careers, may lack the broader personal and professional skill set required for effective delivery and implementation of analysis, going on to suggest that if they do attempt to deliver, this may lead to the devaluing of the feedback system.

Such findings lead to interesting discussions regarding the competencies required to deliver effectively, and who should deliver directly to the athletes. As it stands, empirical research suggests that players seem to prefer delivery from coaches, rather than analysts, which formulates their view on the discipline. In accordance with this, only 13% of analysts will deliver directly to players, and the remaining falling directly to coaches (Wright et al., 2013, 2016). This represents a very small proportion of analysts delivering directly, but given that athletes have directly reported that their perceptions and value placed on analysis directly correlates with who is delivering and their competence to do so, it cannot be ignored. Upskilling and education for analyst's professional career development (including direct athlete delivery) is covered elsewhere in this book, which coupled with excellent degrees, courses and development opportunities externally, may help bring more analysts to the fore of delivery, as proficiency and confidence grow. Whether delivering or not, the performance analyst is a key gatekeeper to the translation of messages for practice as they hold core responsibility for creating, cleaning and visualising core messages. This is done in tandem with coaches, with the same research suggesting that 90% of analysts directly discuss their work with coaches before delivery is undertaken by either party.

Perceptions: Analysts

Hugely positive views regarding the use of analysis have been uncovered by the existing action research reviewed thus far, but none of that would be possible without the analysts themselves. Facilitating analysis provision for coaches and athletes is a time consuming and labour-intensive role, often involving considerable hours to collect, code, analyse and deliver insights. The role of the performance analyst is therefore critical to the successful implementation of the discipline to help better inform and educate decision making in sports. Despite that importance, the availability of analysts varies considerably throughout different sports and countries as earlier discussed in the research of Painczyk et al,(2017) and Andersen et al. (2022). Without an analyst responsibility to produce data and outputs for the discipline, if at all, falls to coaches, whilst with an analyst, the role becomes ever more important and embedded. It is critical then that in understanding the role analysis plays that we critically consider the analysts themselves and the pressures and roles placed upon them.

Analysts perceptions of their own job role were established by Wright et al. (2013), having undertaken action research to survey elite football club analysts. Whilst this sample is representative of only one sport, the results are largely generalisable, given the similarity in role clarity for the majority of analysts, across different sporting codes. Analysts confirmed that they feel significant pressures and the need to work long hours in order to meet the demands of the job, often perhaps not remunerated accordingly for these hours. Further skill set requirements include sport specific knowledge alongside awareness and implementation of developing external data sources. Having already convened multiple sources together to prepare for delivery back to end users, there is then a need to communicate information and land messages, with failure to do this effectively being detrimental to learning. The majority (73%) of analysts in Wright et al.'s (2013) study suggest that analysis does not lead feedback sessions, whilst only 13% of analysts themselves deliver directly to players (Wright et al., 2016), leading us to suggest that whilst the role and worth of the discipline is cemented, the trust in analysts to directly deliver this is not yet matching, with the head of the programme, coaches, remaining the predominant deliverers.

A core facet of the analyst's perceptions on their own role is their place within the team and the relationships that they build with those immediately around them. Francis et al. (2015) discussed the notion of trust, discovering that analysts working in high performance settings feel a need to initiate, foster and consolidate professional relationships. Critical as an area of applied expertise, this suggests that an analyst must not only be technically good at their role but also possess desirable characteristics to build and cement authentic relationships with other sporting professionals in a bid to gain trust, and to fit in. Bateman and Jones (2019) discussed the coach-analyst relationship in detail in professional football finding that self-management and professional relationships are critical to a successful relationship, whilst also reiterating the need to fit in. Using the COMPASS Model, their research uncovered that analysts seek to maintain significantly high standards to help maintain these relationships, though this does bring added pressures to deliver under tight timescales. Reflecting on a personal journey to becoming an analyst, Butterworth and Turner (2014) report the importance of quality interpersonal relationships to professional practice and the need for analysts to proactively engage with opportunities in multiple sports to broaden knowledge and network, in turn helping for future roles. Served in detail elsewhere in this book, the development and maintenance of these good relationships is complex and requires a significant investment into the understanding and development of a micro political literacy.

Self-reporting on their role, analysts in Nicholls et al. (2019) researched the most popular implementation areas of analysis in Olympic sports, finding that video analysis is used most commonly, followed by detailed performance profiling work. This is common place in other non-Olympic sports too, with football analysts reporting video analysis as a key component of their roles (Jones et al., 2020), and the increasing prevalence of data analytics evolving into the analysis sphere. That data analysis must be kept up to date though, with those in Nicholls' study reporting that data analysis and profiling must be kept fresh to enable coaches to approach with questions, and the analyst to respond accordingly with data. Universally accepted as important yes, but bringing further pressures to the role of an analyst.

Analysts also report that they must carefully consider their learning environments, with Reeves and Roberts (2013) research in elite youth football citing the importance. The learning environment is the diverse physical location and culture which considers contextual factors as learning takes place. Often used as an alternative to classroom, which has more traditional connotations, the learning environment encompasses culture, ethos and characteristics including the interaction of people. Analysts therefore are responsible for this, with the physical, contextual and cultural environment having to be considered each time alongside suitable technologies to implement. The paper also reports the need for analysts to learn professional judgement about when to question coaches and when to adopt new technologies. These are not easy concepts and bring about complexities for any analyst, especially those new into their career and learning their craft. The perceptions of the analyst community reviewed here therefore confirm the positive role the discipline plays, but also highlights barriers which they must overcome and the incredibly important role analysts have in devising analysis content for the betterment of performance.

Quantitative Evidence and Efficacy of Analysis

Though sparse in number, there are limited empirical sources which do provide quantitative evidence of the actual impact of analysis on performance outcomes. Racket sports research dominates here, with Brown and Hughes (1995) studying the differing effects of qualitative and quantitative feedback in junior squash players, who favoured the former. Murray et al. (1998) then investigated the use of analysis in aiding feedback to elite and sub-elite squash players and monitored its effect on performance level. They found that after an eight-week intervention programme which included computerised analysis of both data and video, that significant differences were apparent in many of the variables studied. Specifically, the number of errors dropped dramatically for sub-elite players, while for elite players there were still marginal gains, though not as evident as the sub elite group. That said, given the small margins by which elite performances can be won and lost, this still represents a very interesting finding.

Further empirical evidence comes from Jenkins et al.'s (2007) study into the effectiveness of analysis in a sub-elite netball team. They found descriptive quantitative increases in performance level as analysis was introduced, though these findings were not statistically significant. Also undertaking qualitative questionnaires as part of the same study, the authors correlated positive views from the players involved as to the value and place of analysis. In football, Olsen and Larsen (1997) earlier found that the use of computerised analysis for the international side Norway, significantly enhanced their on-pitch performances and allowed them to maximise their otherwise limited resources to compete with the best teams in the world, notably involving wins over England in the 1994 World Cup and Brazil in the 1998 iteration. Egil Olsen, the then manager of the side is quoted as stating that whilst analysis might not be pretty, it works. Additional works in Gaelic Football by Martin et al. (2004) also discovered improvements, with reduced errors and accuracy of free kicks some of the notable positive changes in play, with the intervention of performance analysis seen to impact that.

Towards a Consensus

Reviewing the perceptions of coaches, athletes and analysts towards the value of performance analysis helps lead us towards positive agreements regarding its usefulness in practice and the role it plays in enhancing results. Coaches naturally forget and mis-interpret events from matches and training, and so need an aid to help fill the information deficit. The technologically rich discipline of performance analysis helps with this, and coaches confirm through these action research studies, the important role it plays in helping deliver enhanced outcomes for performers. Subsequently, those athletes themselves also report the efficacious use of performance analysis, shown to help increase engagement and interaction with learning in some demographic groups.

With advanced technologies further aiding retention and learning, in specifically designed learning environments, it is the analysts who are largely responsible for them, and they who come under increasing pressures to deliver outstanding analysis support. Their role is imperative delivering outstanding insights into the coaching process, though the work takes considerable time, effort and emotional investment. These take time to develop with early career analysts requiring emotional and moral support in their development, especially regarding the building and maintenance of critical working relationships.

Further evidence from quantitative studies also points to the empirically proven worth of analysis practice, with early racket sports research especially stating the importance of the discipline in enhancing practice. Driven by objective data and video evidence to help back up, the effectiveness of the discipline plays an important role in developing more effective feedback mechanisms and helping fill an information deficit. Simultaneously, the efficacious use of performance analysis is also shown to help increase engagement and interaction with learning in some demographic groups, whilst allowing others to maximise resources and compete at a higher than expected level, due to analysis support.

It is fair to summarise that the use of analysis is widely received with praise and positivity, with consistent messaging regarding the constructive impact it has on performance outcomes. Though we nod towards a consensus of positivity, a one-size-fits-all, universally encompassing positive approach to analysis will never be achieved and should not be desired, such are the varying contextual, cultural and environmental factors that affect sporting performance. It is those factors that make the sports we watch and work in so engaging, deep rooted in creativity. What this consensus does point towards though, is the role analysis has to play and the ongoing impact it has. And so, we see through critical research insight and quantitative studies, the cascading impact of analysis to impact upon performance; from analyst construction, to coach interpretation to athlete implementation; the analysis domino effect.

Concluding Remarks

Objective and unprejudiced, performance analysis plays an important role in the ongoing development of athletes. In research studies and also practitioner conversations, questions have been asked previously which attain towards trying to consider if the discipline actually works. Rhetorical evidence suggests an overwhelming positive air about the discipline, with clear links to pedagogical principles and developmental learning. The most eminent of these findings have the potential to be impactful on future delivery for coach, athlete and analyst education. Whilst a one-size-fits-all approach will never be attained, important lessons can be learnt about the implementation of analysis, including important practical considerations for current and aspiring analysts alike. Absorbing the amassing number of action research studies in the area with coaches, athletes and analysts alike, we can now more confidently say, *yes*, performance analysis does work and is an undeniably positive addition to the coaching process.

References

Almeida, J., Sarmento, H., Kelly, S., & Travassos, B. (2019). Coach decision making in futsal: From preparation to competition. *International Journal of Performance Analysis in Sport, 19*(3), 1–13.

Andersen, L.W., Francis, J.W., & Bateman, M. (2022). Danish association football coaches' perception of performance analysis. *International Journal of Performance Analysis in Sport, 22*(1), 149–173.

Bampouras, T.M., Cronin, C., & Miller, P.K. (2012). Performance analytic processes in elite sport practice: An exploratory investigation of the perspectives of a sport scientist, coach and athlete. *International Journal of Performance Analysis in Sport, 12*(2), 468–483.

Bateman, M., & Jones, G. (2019). Strategies for maintaining the coach–analyst relationship within professional football utilizing the COMPASS model: The performance analyst's perspective. *Frontiers in Psychology, 10*, 2064.

Brown, D., & Hughes, M. (1995). The effectiveness of quantitative and qualitative feedback on performance in squash. In T. Reilly, M. Hughes, & A. Lees (Eds.), *Science and racket sports* (pp. 232–237). London: E & FN Spon.

Butterworth, A.D., & Turner, D.J. (2014). Becoming a performance analyst: Auto-ethnographic reflections on agency, and facilitated transformational growth. *Reflective Practice, 15*(5), 552–562.

Butterworth, A.D., Turner, D.J., & Johnstone, J. (2012). Coaches perceptions of the potential use of performance analysis in badminton. *International Journal of Performance Analysis in Sport, 12*(2), 452–467.

De Martin Silva, L., & Francis, J.W. (2020). "It is like a little journey": Deaf international futsal players' and coaches' experiences in collaborative blended learning. *International Sport Coaching Journal, 8*(2), 183–196.

Fernandez-Echeverria, C., Mesquita, I., Conejero, M., & Moreno, M.P. (2019). Perceptions of elite volleyball players on the importance of match analysis during the training process. *International Journal of Performance Analysis in Sport, 19*(1), 49–64.

Francis, J., & Jones, G. (2014). Elite rugby union players perceptions of performance analysis. *International Journal of Performance Analysis in sport, 14*(1), 188–207.

Francis, J., Molnar, G., Donovan, M., & Peters, D. (2015). Trust within a high performance sport: A performance analyst's perspective. *Journal of Sports Sciences, 33*(Suppl. 1), 47–48.

Franks, I.M., & Miller, G. (1991). Training coaches to observe and remember. *Journal of Sports Sciences, 9*(3), 285–297.

Groom, R., & Cushion, C. (2004). Coaches perceptions of the use of video analysis: A case study. *Insight, 7*(3), 56–58.

Groom, R., & Cushion, C.J. (2005). Using of video based coaching with players: A case study. *International Journal of Performance Analysis in Sport, 5*(3), 40–46.

Groom, R., Cushion, C., & Nelson, L. (2011). The delivery of video-based performance analysis by England youth soccer coaches: Towards a grounded theory. *Journal of Applied Sport Psychology, 23*(1), 16–32.

Guitierrez-Aguilar, O., Montoya-Fernandez, M., Fernandez-Romero, J.J., & Saavedra-Garcia, A.M. (2016). Analysis of time out use in handball and its influence on the game performance. *International Journal of Performance Analysis in Sport, 16*(1), 1–11.

Horne, S. (2013). The role of performance analysis in elite netball competition structures. In D. Peters & P. O'Donoghue (Eds.), *Performance analysis of sport IX* (pp. 30–37). London: Routledge.

Jenkins, E.R., Morgan, L., & O'Donoghue, P. (2007). A case study into the effectiveness of computerised match analysis and motivational videos within the coaching of a league netball team. *International Journal of Performance Analysis in Sport, 7*(2), 59–80.

Jones, D., Rands, S., & Butterworth, A.D. (2020). The use and perceived value of telestration tools in elite football. *International Journal of Performance Analysis in Sport, 20*(3), 373–388.

Kraak, W., Magwa, Z., & Terblanche, E. (2018). Analysis of South African semi-elite rugby head coaches' engagement with performance analysis. *International Journal of Performance Analysis in Sport, 18*(2), 350–366.

Laird, P., & Waters, L. (2008). Eye witness recollection of sports coaches. *International Journal of Performance Analysis in Sport, 8*(1), 76–84.

Loo, J.K., Francis, J., & Bateman, M. (2020). Athletes' and coaches' perspectives of performance analysis in women's sports in Singapore. *International Journal of Performance Analysis in Sport, 20*(6), 960–981.

Martin, D., Cassidy, D., & O'Donoghue, P. (2004). *The effectiveness of performance analysis in elite Gaelic football.* Paper presented at the 5th world congress of performance analysis of sport, Belfast, May 2004.

Martin, D., Swanton, A., Bradley, J.J., McGrath, D., & Bradley, J.J. (2018). The use, integration and perceived value of performance analysis to professional and amateur Irish coaches. *International Journal of Sports Science and Coaching, 13*(4), 520–532.

Mayes, A., O'Donoghue, P.G., Garland, J., & Davidson, A. (2009) *The use of performance analysis and internet video streaming during elite netball preparation.* Paper presented at the 3rd international workshop of the international society of performance analysis of sport, Lincoln, April 2009.

Middlemas, S., & Harwood, C. (2017). No place to hide: Football players' and coaches' perceptions of the psychological factors influencing video feedback. *Journal of Applied Sport Psychology, 30*(1), 23–44.

Mooney, R., Corley, G., Godfrey, A., Osborough, C., Newell, J., Quinlan, L.R., & OLaighin, G. (2016). Analysis of swimming performance: Perceptions and practices of US-based swimming coaches. *Journal of Sports Sciences, 34*(11), 997–1005.

Moreno-Perla, M., Moreno, A., Garcia-Gonzalez, L., Urena, A., Hernandez, C., & Del Villar, F. (2016). An intervention based on video feedback and questionning to improve tactical knowledge in expert female volleyball players. *Perceptual and Motor Skills, 122*(3), 911–932.

Murray, S., Maylor, D., & Hughes, M. (1998). A preliminary investigation into the provision of computerised analysis feedback to elite squash players. In A. Lees, I. Maynard, M. Hughes, & T. Reilly (Eds.), *Science and racket sports II* (pp. 235–240). London: E and FN Spon.

Nelson, L., Potrac, P., & Groom, R. (2014). Receiving video-based feedback in elite ice-hockey: A players perspective. *Sport, Education and Society, 1*(1), 19–40.

Nicholls, S.B., James, N., Bryant, E., & Wells, J. (2019). The implementation of performance analysis and feedback within Olympic sport: The performance analyst's perspective. *International Journal of Sports Science & Coaching, 14*(1), 63–71.

O'Donoghue, P. (2010). *Research methods for sports performance analysis.* London: Routledge.

Olsen, E., & Larsen, O. (1997). Use of match analysis by coaches. In T. Reilly, J. Bangsbo, & M. Williams (Eds.), *Science and football III* (pp. 209–220). London: E & FN Spon.

Painczyk, H., Hendricks, S., & Kraak, W. (2017). Utilisation of performance analysis among Western Province Rugby Union club coaches. *International Journal of Performance Analysis in Sport, 17*(6), 1057–1072.

Reeves, M.J., & Roberts, S.J. (2013). Perceptions of performance analysis in elite youth football. *International Journal of Performance Analysis in Sport, 13*(1), 200–211.

Wright, C., Atkins, S., & Jones, B. (2012). An analysis of elite coaches' engagement with performance analysis services (match, notational and technique). *International Journal of Performance Analysis in Sport, 12*(2), 436–451.

Wright, C., Atkins, S., Jones, B., & Todd, J. (2013). The role of performance analysts within the coaching process: Performance Analysts Survey 'The role of performance analysts in elite football club settings.' *International Journal of Performance Analysis, 13*(1), 240–261.

Wright, C., Carling, C., Lawlor, C., & Collins, D. (2016). Elite football player engagement with performance analysis. *International Journal of Performance Analysis in Sport, 16*(3), 1007–1032.

8

CAREER DEVELOPMENT AND PROFESSIONAL LITERACY

Andrew Butterworth

Introduction

Gaining employment in the performance analysis industry is notoriously competitive. It is well documented and publicised that the number of budding analysts and subsequently applicants to roles far outweighs the volume of positions on offer. Often, hundreds apply for a single role, making the shortlisting and interview processes for employers an exceptionally difficult task. It is undoubtedly a more difficult process though for the applicants themselves (you reading this book), which can often result in a disheartening or disappointing outcome. For those with existing qualifications or experience, navigating the process and trying to understand what you require to be successful in future applications can be difficult. Equally so, starting out from scratch and considering a future career in the industry can be daunting given the existing extreme popularity and competitive nature of working in applied performance analysis.

The good news is that there are a growing number of performance analysis roles in the professional sphere, as the popularity and importance of the role continues to be embedded. Traditionally roles were associated and entwined predominantly with mainstream popular team sports such as football and rugby union, and so the number of roles until more recent times has been somewhat limited. Though now, there are a much wider variety of roles on offer as the discipline continues to evolve and develop into a mainstay of the IDT and a key component of the complex coaching process. The welcome emergence of professionalism in more women's sports and the advent of professional leagues in football, rugby and netball to name but a few, is excellent news not only for the sports themselves, but for the analysis community, with full time roles now on offer in each of these settings. Academy and junior age group analysis positions are also becoming more common as organisations seek to engrain analysis within their

DOI: 10.4324/9781003226659-8

pathway athletes from an early age which again result in more advertised opportunities for prospective analysts. Individual sports, especially those such as tennis, badminton and squash are also investing more in analysis support, and so roles are emerging there, as they are too in the long-awaited materialisation of more roles in para-sport settings. Our use of data, analytics and programming software in practical analysis roles has developed also, and so there are many more specialist roles emerging in these spheres for candidates with the right skill set.

This emergence and the continually growing field of performance analysis is indeed good news, but the roles will continue to be competitive given the continuing popularity of analysis as a prospective career route. For those starting out and considering a career path in this field, or those with experience but yet to gain their desired employment, this predicament can be daunting and sometimes off-putting. Therefore, this chapter seeks to provide insight into how aspiring analysts can enhance their employment prospects, drawing upon multiple different routes into the industry. There are a number of steps and professional competencies that prospective employees can seek to gain in an attempt to enhance their prospects of employment. These steps are discussed in this chapter, drawn from peer-reviewed literature, insights from the authors' experience as an analyst and recruiter, alongside advice and guidance from those who currently work as analysts, many of whom are in recruiting positions. There is no set way into gaining an analysis job, with those who already work in the industry coming from many varied backgrounds, though what is common, is that early applied experience is vital for future employment. Here, we'll examine tips and potential steps for enhancing your practice as an analyst in the real world, gaining a resulting competitive advantage in your next application.

'It's About Who You Know'

You'll be hard pressed to have a conversation with anyone working in the performance analysis industry, without them making at least a fleeting mention of this. Often referred to as three degrees of separation, it is true that the professional network of performance analysts is close knit, and indeed everyone does seem to know everyone. That might be just to make small talk on the gantry on match days and check the easiest route down to the changing rooms, or some relationships are much stronger with numerous examples of very good friends working in the industry, perhaps those who have been through university and lived together, before going on to work for rival clubs. Further still, others will end up as groomsmen or bridesmaids at weddings, and remain lifelong friends, not least since they know *exactly* when to ask the DJ to drop Mr Brightside.

Joking asides, it is true that forming strong relationships in the industry is one of the most important skills for a budding analyst to develop, and too for those already working in the industry but seeking to progress further. The ability to network with those who work in elite roles, perhaps one that you are aspiring to attain in the future, can be a considerable help to not only gain contacts, but also to build confidence in your abilities. On the surface networking might seem easy, in that you make a connection, send a message and that is that, but it is far from that simple. There are multiple layers to consider, especially in an ever scrutinous social media-driven world.

Social media sites Twitter and LinkedIn are the two used most often by those seeking to connect to those already in the industry. There are some outstanding analysts and organisations on both of these sites who are regularly sharing content, ideas and tips. Some are more open than others, and these ideas and content in itself can be an excellent way to build your own knowledge. Webinars, 1--2-1 chats and mentoring and general chats are also offered out here, all of which should be considered as excellent networking opportunities. As a starting point, creating yourself a profile on each of these sites, and following or connecting with those in positions is a terrific resource.

However, for those on the receiving end, yet another connection on LinkedIn or another follow on Twitter can often seem meaningless, and indeed if you are seeking to network with a view to making a real connection with someone, a *cold* follow is not likely to lead to anything more. If you really want to make a mark, to really be noticed and start speaking to professionals working in the field, then be bold and start a conversation with those people. That said, "Can you give me a job please" is probably not your best conversation starter, and so you should think carefully about the message you are trying to convey, what you are trying to achieve and the professionalism with which it comes across. Introduce yourself, who you are, where you aspire to be and how you intend to make it there. Be really bold and ask if they would have time for a short conversation, or offer to buy them a coffee next time they are in your area for a game (free coffee always goes down a treat!). But keep it short. Long messages will not be read, and the core message will be lost amongst the noise. Make sure that your writing and professional stature come across too, with those with poorer spelling, grammar and structure, tend not to make it past the *seen* or *read* stage and instead get safely stored in the recycle bin. And so, if you are going to reach out, do it with purpose, conviction and professionalism, after all; this is the first impression you are making.

If you do make a connection, it is likely that the professional on the receiving end will click onto your profile, out of natural human curiosity. And so, do not get caught out (like many have before you), instead ensure that your profile conveys the message that you want it to. Consider what your handle (e.g. your @ username) actually is, what your profile picture is, your header photo and you limited characters bio information. @Lesta4Lyf (no endorsements or insult supported to that particular handle if it exists) intoxicated pictures from your birthday or defamatory remarks in a bio are not going to be suited. Neither are Twitter accounts which are laden with expletive riddled tweets or re-tweets. All of these things, no matter how small they seem, will convey a message to the reader, and so think professional, courteous and well-mannered.

As and when you do make connections, make the most of them. Ask those people how they got to where they did, what they look for when recruiting, any tips for what you can do. If you're feeling particularly bold, ask if there is an opportunity for you to shadow them or someone else in their department for a day, and then make the most of that too. If you have a guest lecture at your university or attend a conference, go up and make a real human connection with the speakers. Don't just file out of the room (physical or virtual) having not made sure that the speaker knows your name. This is perhaps the most difficult of all, and exceptionally daunting as your heart beats out of your chest approaching the analyst of your own supported team at a conference to mumble out your name and ask if you can buy them a coffee to chat about analysis (personal experience!). But it is a situation worth embracing and braving. All of these interactions will positively impact your future career. Months, years or decades later when you apply for a job with that person, your name, your interaction and your boldness might just stimulate a reminder for them, triggering a previous encounter, which might just serve you well.

Amongst all this through, what is not true, is that it is simply knowing people in the industry that will gain you a job role. You also have to be good at what you do, really good. You're also going to need suitable qualifications, applied experiences, know how to write a strong cover letter and interview well, alongside the ability to effectively communicate messages to a plethora of people. Luckily, this chapter is intended to help you do just that.

Entering the Industry

Formal Education

There is no set way by which to enter into the performance analysis industry, with multiple options available including via experience, short courses, college courses, accreditations, apprenticeships and higher education degrees. That said, expectations are changing as the industry continues to become ever more professional and more formal training opportunities emerge and the essential criteria on job applications continue to grow.

As the discipline first started to gain popularity and began to become a more formal role in sports science teams, there were no formal qualifications available and most analysts will have learned directly on the job using transferable skills. As the role popularised, those wishing to work as an analyst will have typically studied sport at college or school through their GCSE and A-Level's, alongside other subjects of personal interest. Beyond this, they will likely have gone on to study a broad sport science or sports studies degree, which may have perhaps included modules on performance analysis (though likely taught by a coach or biomechanist), before going on to specialise and focus independent study projects in the discipline, if supervision expertise allowed. Beyond this, those who had developed a significant desire to work in the industry may have gone on to the first UK-based MSc programme, which was developed and taught by the then University of Wales Institute, Cardiff (Now Cardiff Metropolitan University) in 2003. This offered the first real taught provision of performance analysis in the UK (and perhaps globally) and continues today.

Now, the performance analysis education landscape is significantly changed, with a vast number of universities recognising the growing importance and popularity and so developing taught content and research opportunities. There are now at least five UK-based undergraduate degrees in performance analysis. In addition, of the hundreds of different sport-related degrees, a huge number now offer performance analysis modules and pathways, representing again the popularity and importance of the discipline. Furthermore, developing at an even quicker pace are postgraduate degrees in performance analysis, with some twinned alongside applied placements such as the Applied Performance Analysis MSc at Loughborough University which started in 2021. Such has been the proliferation of new MSc and MRes programmes in performance analysis in recent years, the last count in the United Kingdom stands at 14, with others also in development. Multiple courses of course bring competition, and students now have a number of important considerations to make when electing where to go, including location, facilities, professional links and staff expertise.

As such, the *typical* route into a performance analysis job now is to undertake such education courses alongside practical experience, before seeking a role. This represents a huge change for the industry as a highly skilled and formally trained workforce emerges with recognised qualifications. This is speaking predominantly about the UK market, with only a very small number of opportunities and formal courses existing elsewhere around the globe. Some enter immediately after school age, with others retraining at a later age and learning as they enter into a new industry. Many of these degrees embed additional qualifications and certifications in product use too, and as such the quality of degrees is now generally high, as too are the graduates. This is also reflected in job descriptions, with a relevant undergraduate degree, bespoke MSc, and considerable applied experience using multiple systems now commonplace as essential criteria. This said, there are also opportunities, especially for those in data analyst roles, who often come from mathematics or physics backgrounds, and reapply their skillset in a different professional context.

Further, there are now approved level five apprenticeship standards for performance analysis, and so it is likely soon that universities will start to offer the delivery of these to clubs, who will likely be keen and utilise the levy money they are obliged to pay by the government. With unpaid internships and funded placements having been the two popular methods for student recruitment and experience in the industry so far, perhaps apprenticeships will be next, albeit in a more structured and legal way with considerable configuration and planning embedded in these offers behind the scenes.

For those starting out, given the thousands of students who graduate every year with formal performance analysis education and the stiff competition for jobs, this represents a myriad of options and sometimes confusion or concern. Given the essential criteria on most jobs now state a degree, many will opt for the formal higher education options. Though that is not to say it is the only way, with many analysts succeeding through other means too. The remainder of this chapter will focus on those additional means by which you might help yourself become more employable, regardless of if you are in or out of formal higher education, to make the most of prospective opportunities and attempt to stand out in a crowded industry whilst developing your craft as an analyst.

In addition to formal higher education courses, there are also a number of other additional avenues by which prospective or current analysts can sharpen their craft. Numerous different short courses, additional qualifications and accreditations are now on offer for analysts to aid their ongoing professional development, as too are conference and mentoring opportunities. Here, with no direct endorsements to any, we'll take a look at some of those and the relative value that they provide to helping enhance career prospects and ongoing professional development.

Making the Most of It

Regardless of which avenue you select, taking that opportunity fully and engaging with the opportunities on offer is vital. Indeed, the importance of this cannot be understated as all too often, those who cite they want to be a performance analyst or want to become a better performance analyst do not actively engage and take steps towards achieving that, instead seemingly assuming that some form of osmosis will occur. Of course, this is not true to all, and there are many who do take proactive steps towards enhancing their prospects. But it does seem that there a number who 'coast' through with no real drive towards improvement, with Butterworth and Turner (2014) noting that some do not seem at all willing to engage deeply with learning, instead remaining in a comfort zone where meaningful personal growth and transformation cannot happen. And so, the additional opportunities outlined here are intended to help you avoid that, moving yourself out of your immediate comfort zone towards consequential professional growth.

Further qualifications and accreditations do not necessarily imply competence or ability, yet seemingly will help you get job roles. If selected carefully and engaged with fully, given the growing number of requirements appearing on job descriptions, additional qualifications or accreditations to undertake which contain applied delivery will help your ongoing professional development. Selecting which to undertake though is not as straightforward, with a plethora of different options from multiple different organisations or individuals now available.

Short Courses and Certification

In addition to formal higher education courses, there also now exist a number of short courses and certifications in performance analysis. Whilst there is no set definition for a short course, general consensus agrees that there should be a series of lessons or lectures on a certain topic, rather than a single one, to be classed as a course. It is important here too to consider the *certification* element, which could be as simple as a home-made PDF certificate, or more formal official documents which attests to a status or level of achievement. The latter would suggest some form of assessment, which is infrequently part of any of the courses on offer, instead most opt for an attendance-based certification. Given the huge number of courses now on offer, how these are approached should be done carefully, and the value attributed to them weighed up in a cost-benefit manner.

Initially, potential candidates should consider who it is that is offering the course, their reputation and the people who sit behind it. Those with considerable expertise and experience in the industry will bring significant value to a short course, and likely be in a position to share stories, hints and tips about their time and skills. Major players in the short course market include the English Institute of Sport (EIS), who offer their very well regarded 'Skills 4 Performance' series in a number of sport sciences, not just analysis, or Steve Ingham's 'Supporting Champions' courses again in multiple disciplines. The EIS offer, though not run since the global pandemic, is competitive with an application process and is highly coveted, offering an immersive learning experience with highly experienced practitioners in Olympic and Paralympic sport. Steve Ingham meanwhile offers insight into the role itself, but importantly also into the soft skills and personal attributes that sit alongside the techniques and technology expertise.

This previous experience and direction of those running or involved in the courses should be a consideration too, and if your desire is to work within Olympic programmes, then this might be a critical offer to target your involvement with. Those who have had, or still hold similar jobs to the one you have in mind may be very beneficial to you, perhaps the Professional Football Scouts Association (PFSA) course might be best if you wish to work in recruitment or talent ID, as too might the United Kingdom Coaching Certificate (UKCC) course in scouting. For data analysis, perhaps the STATS match and performance analysis course might be best suited, given the focus and likely experience of the practitioners delivering.

You should also research and consider the learning method, trying to ensure that there are opportunities on the course for interaction and applied learning, not just passive remote based dictation, in a 'talk and chalk' style. The importance of a course might lie in the skills and knowledge gained, but it might also lie in the communication, question and networking opportunities, if they exist. Having the chance to interact with both those running the course and those on it, reflective practice and feedback opportunities are important considerations.

In addition to these, the many technology companies discussed in detail earlier in this book now offer a series of courses or loosely termed qualifications in using their products too. The major companies have invested significant time, human resource and technology into developing remote-based learning platforms for using their products, driven by newly formed education teams. Most do have a form of assessment by way of an analysis task to show competency, with some offering feedback and 1-2-1 tips if required to further drive improvements. Better still, if you are a university or college student, these courses are becoming more commonly included in your studies, as part of booming contracts for software and hardware. If you are not on such an educational pathway, the costs are not typically extortionate and so provide relative value for money. In selecting which if any to embark on, again think about the role you are aiming for, and target the provider whose software is utilised most widely in that sport. For those keeping their options open as to which sport to enter into, there may of course be value in undertaking more than one, and provide a holistic understanding of the software on offer. If money is a constraint, then there are some excellent video tutorials online and free resources offered on social media by prominent analysts, which coupled with a short free trial period of a chosen software, might be just the spark needed to drive further exploration into the potential career path.

What is perhaps lacking mostly in the educational market at the moment though is the equivalent hardware certifications. With Apple Mac still dominating the performance analysis sphere, and increasing numbers of evolving technologies, there is a huge array of sometimes complicated technology required. To live stream, provide stats and video on the bench in near real time for example needs significant infrastructure investment and set up, alongside networking knowledge around IP addresses, network protocols and sharing settings. Quite often, this learning comes on the job, through experience and through shadowing or working with elite analysts in situ. Some do offer an introduction to this, but a focussed course in and around these elements would significantly benefit the industry as it grows.

Coaching Qualifications

On many analysis job adverts, an additional desirable (occasionally essential) criteria will list a recognised level two or above coaching qualification in the sport. These courses are desired as they help deliver sport specific knowledge and tactics which may prove useful in practice, especially for those perhaps starting to work in a less familiar sport. Initial theory will provide understanding and appreciation of the coaching process which underpins the analysis work, and also stimulate thought about the context in which analysis is delivered and the complexities involved. Many courses on the UKCC register now mandate that there is a focus and sometimes practice on analysis (and other disciplines too) to help educate coaches as to the worth of the discipline in their practice, inverting this relationship provides considerable value for the analysis community. Those other disciplines will also prove valuable as the knowledge may help build IDT underpinning and work for the analyst.

If an analyst cannot deliver their message and land it with the end user, much of their work will be void. With that in mind, the communication and relationship building aspects of coaching course will also sit analysts in good stead for future job roles and impacting fully with their work. Learning environments, styles and feedback strategies will also all be considered in coaching situ too, which again will serve as useful context for an analyst seeking to operate in this messy and socially derived environment. Cost can be an impeding factor to these courses, as too can frequency and location, but where possible, the courses do provide a valuable resource for developing analysis and coaching craft with a deepened appreciation.

Accreditations

Where many other sports sciences have accrediting or professional bodies, for example the United Kingdom Strength and Conditioning Association (UKSCA) or Sport and Exercise Nutrition Register (SENR), the same cannot be said for performance analysis. In other sciences, these accreditations provide assurance to employers that they have met and evidenced certain standards in different elements of the profession, which in turn subsequently helps in the selection of suitably qualified candidates to fill vacancies. The British Association of Sport and Exercise Sciences (BASES) also offers various accreditations in sport and exercise science, but requires applicants to be existing members and there is no focus on performance analysis, though work is in progress to change that with the advent of the BASES Performance Analysis Special Interest Group. That currently leaves our discipline with no formal accreditation available, with it not yet benefitting from a thorough competency based and fulfilling worthwhile accreditation.

The International Society of Performance Analysis in Sport (ISPAS) does offer a form of accreditation, allowing those who work as performance analysts with relevant experience to apply. The application process invites applicants to self-select the level at which they wish to apply for, based upon their own interpretation of the guidance notes and how many years work they have accumulated. Applicants pay the fee online before then writing a letter outlining their experience without the need to attach any evidence, which is rewarded by a confirmatory email if the panel agree. This system is a little problematic in that it predominantly rewards the number of years' experience and level at which an applicant has worked, rather than the skill set needed to work as an analyst.

Once accredited, analysts will benefit from small book discounts, reduced licence costs for Focus X2 software (though that is all but outdated from the market now) and discounted fees at ISPAS events, in addition to being able to add their status to their CVs. What it does not offer is help, mentoring, continual professional development (CPD) opportunities, networking or sustained support to ongoing development, which come with more established accreditations in the other sport sciences. Despite this, many jobs will still list the ISPAS accreditations as criteria on job descriptions, though this is probably most likely as there are no other viable alternatives, and it is exceptionally unlikely that a decision to shortlist, interview or appoint will be based upon having the accreditation or not.

Moving forwards, there is a need for a more thorough and rewarding accreditation scheme in performance analysis, which is based upon a skills-based and competency award, cognisant of the technologically driven and rapidly developing industry. An accreditation which offers mentoring and support alongside continual development opportunities and learning schemes would be welcome, and further help analysts develop their work and continually progress. In time, this may change, with some conversations already happening and developments in line to progress this area of professional practice, though as it stands the accreditation options are severely limited. That change though will take significant time, human resource and dedication, alongside help from the wider performance analysis community.

Webinars, Guest Speakers and Conferences

Aside from excellent lunches and the occasional post-event drink, performance analysis conferences can provide valued learning opportunities and networking. Depending the focus, conferences can provide multiple speakers from a single sporting industry, or a variety from different sports. Targeting your attendance at those events which have speakers holding roles you wish to pursue, or those whose work you admire, will likely be a key influencing decision. When there, networking with others, drawing influence from the presentations and connecting with the speakers are key remits to try and achieve. The drawback though is often the prohibitive cost and far flung locations. Single-day events can be anywhere in the region of £100+, whilst longer events will fetch many times that, not to mention any which might be hosted abroad. A move to more online conferences and virtual event has been apparent more recently, which has helped with attendance and engagement, whilst also enabling a wider audience to reach the events.

In seeking any positives from the global pandemic, one such might be the increased efficiency of a virtual workplace and advent of more such remote learning opportunities online. The first lockdown in 2020 saw a flurry of excellent webinars and learning opportunities for budding analysts, with professionals in the field recognising the impact and disruption to education, and wanting to give something back. As the next newest webinar appeared on social media, whilst some might have been thinking 'Not another webinar' (which snappily became the authors' own webinar series title, offering free 1-2-1 chats for an optional charitable donation), there were undoubtedly some excellent resources, practical sessions, Q&A opportunities and tutorials on offer, many free of charge. Some of those materials and offers are still available, and form an excellent learning resource for many, and so might be considered as a way in which to enhance practice further.

Pre-pandemic, the typical way in which to hear from experts would be through guest lectures at school, college or university. This continues again now, picking up more so as restrictions ease, and provide valuable networking opportunities to engage with. Keen to showcase real-world practice to students, staff seek to utilise their own contacts to bring in experts to showcase their work-flows, tips for practice and hints for employment prospects. Such sessions are critical to your development as an analyst. The rich level of insight that they will undoubtedly provide might just spark an interest, a different perspective, a fresh way of approaching a task, or a gem of information to use in practice. Even if the upcoming speaker is from a sport you are less interested in, attend that session and engage with the speaker. The principles of analysis remain largely steadfast across sports, with the application and focus points different in each, and so attending and seeing analysis from another perspective can be valuable, with ideas to take away and use in your own work. Engagement in other sports also shows willing on applications and job interviews, and is often viewed positively rather than someone with a one sport fixation. Better still, ask a question during the inevitable awkward silences and be the first brave person to speak up, then speak directly to the speaker afterwards, make sure that they know your name and perhaps even be bold and offer to buy them a coffee after the session.

Applied Experience

The biggest weapon an aspiring performance analyst can add to their arsenal is to gain a rich variety of applied experiences in industry. Whilst qualifications, education and courses will help satisfy job description criterion and perhaps place you on a shortlist of potential candidates, your experience in the field in real-life scenarios using technology, interacting with staff and players and an ability to evidence that will get you the job. Experiences may come through a variety of mediums, but may often start with either a work experience or shadowing opportunity, followed by an entry-level analysis role completing vital filming and coding tasks, for use in wider analysis workflows. Whilst these can be somewhat monotonous, they challenge the aspiring analyst to consider the underpinnings of the discipline and provide a greater appreciation for the mechanics that sit beneath the more stimulating analysis tasks and feedback processes. As competencies grow, analysts will be provided with more responsibility and tasks, developing over time in situ with organisational requirements and analysis philosophies.

Historically, sourcing initial experience roles can be a challenge in itself, with the growing popularity of the discipline leading to an overflow of willing candidates keen to start their journey. Many opportunities now will come via internship or placements which may be formalised and pre-agreed with clubs alongside university courses where partnerships with local organisations may be embedded. Whilst this may seem to close the door for those not going to University, that need not be the case. Either in or out of higher education, it is encouraged to be bold, reaching out to prospective organisations and local clubs and challenging oneself in different sports, taking note from the networking section earlier in this chapter. The level at which an experience is available is often a consideration, with many seeking the highest possible club or organisation roles early on.

However, early career analysts should never believe that a club or role is beneath them, it is in fact sometimes those roles which are in lower league clubs or less well funded sports that promote innovation and real professional growth.

The ethics of initial roles is also hotly contested; there have been many developments in the early roles in recent years. Historically, initial experiences were termed as *internships* whereby clubs and organisations would take on willing volunteers, and expect the budding analyst to work extensive hours for little or no remuneration. For many this included any travel costs incurred which could potentially turn expensive. This provided a conundrum, whereby the experience offered was invaluable for future development and potential employment, but the personal and financial cost was dear. Though for clubs, it was perhaps ideal, getting free labour and thinking little if at all, about the analysts' welfare or socio-economic status. Developing rapidly to almost all organisations, internships were common place, though as time further developed and national practice and policy around unpaid internships developed, these started to become more obsolete. Though exceptionally rare, some clubs still do offer out these 'opportunities', whilst it has been pleasing to see that the industry now starts to call out such practices, and continually question the ethics and morals of such practice.

In place of entirely unpaid internships came some paid roles, typically at the national living wage, which did at least recognise the analyst's contribution and role within the club. Soon, placement years emerged as a more popular route, with undergraduate roles as part of a sandwich year, or postgraduate study options becoming utilised more often. For each, an intensive year in industry did (and for some still does) offer an outstanding opportunity to immerse in practice and develop daily alongside experienced staff. Many postgraduate placements were or are embedded alongside taught university courses too, where students balance their time between practical on the job learning, and university academic study. The best outcomes of these are typically from those courses which promote applied learning and entwine the placement hours as part of the core curriculum and assessments, rather than those who are purely classroom-based and theory-centric, which offer little toward the day-to-day practice of the modern analysis role. Further still, some offered to cover tuition fees proving a popular option to limit costs, whilst the latest model appears to be employing students as part time staff, so that they benefit from wider employee benefits such as pension contributions and healthcare, whilst simultaneously finalising studies. With apprenticeship standards now also approved in performance analysis at level five, it will surely not be long before clubs elect to utilise their levy money to fund developmental analysis support this way. The industry has developed well in recent years, and taken on a better ethical and moral stance on the development of new students, though some problems do remain, especially regarding finances, considered more fully in Chapter 9.

Once a role has been secured, making the most of that experience is also key, and not taking it for granted. Those content to do the bear minimum, or those who think that they have made it into the big time by wearing a club tracksuit with your initials on, will likely be found out, and fall by the wayside. Those who invest time in reflection, developing strong working relationships with stakeholders, asking questions and not being afraid to be somewhat vulnerable in doing so, report higher levels of satisfaction, and faster development towards enhanced analysis work practice. Therefore, gaining that applied experience and exposing yourself to multiple environments and many different scenarios will serve well as a tool to develop analysis craft, and later help towards a successful application for that ultimate job role. Those too who step outside of their metaphorical comfort zone, and challenge themselves to work with different sports, different age groups or different environments to that of their desired end goal, tend to develop faster. Exposing yourself to a new environment in a different sport promotes personal growth and encourages reflection on practices, including technology, processes and workflows which may be transferred from one to another, to enhance future practice. Butterworth and Turner (2014) researched this and understood that removing oneself from the comfort zone and being willing to become comfortable with the uncomfortable, embracing uncertainty, brings about rapid growth and transformational change. And so, to the developing analyst now, expose yourself to multiple environments and scenarios, start small and be grateful for an opportunity to shadow or assist, before becoming more embedded, taking on more responsibility and learning to develop craft in analysis workflows. Be humble, take opportunities fully and ensure that reflection and ongoing professional development are central, you are not, and will not for many years, if at all, be a finished product and the perfect analyst.

Application, Interview and Feedback

For any given role, especially the 'popular' ones in sports such as football, anecdotal evidence from those recruiting tells of sometimes 100+ applying for a single role. This represents huge competition for roles and results in difficulties for both applicants and employers. For employers, shortlisting can become a cut-throat process, based upon qualifications as a checklist criterion, whilst quantity and quality of applied experience help drive decisions too. Whittling down a hundred or more applicants to a handful to interview can be tough.

Application

For applicants, having taken the advice in this chapter so far to be in serious contention for employment, the next step is to bring together an outstanding application that makes this shortlist. When initially compiling an application, employers will typically request an updated CV and a cover letter as the first means of registering your interest. The CV acts as a quick reference point for the employer, being able to ascertain personal details alongside prior education and experiences. A CV should never exceed two pages of A4 and should be succinct, simple and to the point ensuring that the most relevant and recent experiences are included prime and centre. Your prospective employer will probably not be so interested in the paper round you held as a 13-year-old or the temporary position at a well-known high-street retailer over the Christmas period one year. The CV should instead make reference to the most relevant experiences and education provisions you have, saving space for the important ones and the opportunity to elaborate in a sentence or two of your role and responsibilities in that environment, rather than listing every role in every sector you have ever held. Where education is concerned, listing every qualification you have individually, the year, the location and the grade isn't required. For GCSE or equivalent, summarise the grades simply and succinctly, whilst still highlighting the important subjects which underpin your knowledge base for this job role, for example;

> Ten GCSE's grades A*-B achieved in 2007, including English, Maths & Science.

As you start to include your more advanced qualifications (e.g. A-Levels and BTECs), do elaborate a little more, but refrain from going into great detail about each, instead maintaining simplicity and clarity of message. For showcasing practical work and prior roles, do include your prior analysis roles, internships, placement years, coaching badges, conference attendance, additional courses and qualifications, but again, hold off on the bar work or mixologist role, after all, in a sphere of 100+ applications, your ability to pour a pint or make an old fashioned, won't be the deciding factor for this analysis role.

A CV need not be two pages (or less) of bland black and white text either. Many aspiring analysts talk about creativity in their role and bringing new ideas, well this is your initial opportunity to show that, and so perhaps consider being bold, and producing a CV which reflects that, with actual design input including colour, imagery and forward-thinking layouts. Please, don't get carried away with MS Paint, but do seriously consider the look and feel of this document, it might be the only first impression you get, and you want to make it a good one. Ruthless as it sounds, shortlisting decisions are made in minutes or seconds, so you need to stand out, you need to highlight the most important experiences early on, to catch the eye and give yourself a fighting chance to ensure that yours doesn't become and safely filed away in the reject pile.

Given the competition for roles, some employers will now utilise an additional or replacement screening of a video introduction. This is an opportunity for them to meet you, see you, understand your character and how you communicate about yourself verbally, not what is written on paper, and will play a huge part in your application. If this is part of an application process, then it is vital that you portray yourself in a positive light, both metaphorically and literally. Attention to detail about where you film this, how you film, and the quality of the end product are vital, after all, you are an analyst who claims to be able to utilise expensive video equipment every day. And so, ensure that you dress smartly and choose an appropriate space including a clean, crisp background to record this.

Light the room accordingly (e.g. not in front of bright windows), make sure that you frame yourself appropriately in the shot and that the audio is clear. If you are using a supporting slide or two, design these professionally and include relevant imagery or logos to show your attention to detail. Don't be afraid to take a few attempts at recording, and edit if needed; use an analysis software to help with this.

The cover letter is your opportunity to expand, and tempt the employer in with a tease of what you can offer, your prior experiences and how that fits with the role on offer. This is also your chance to show your application and evidence of skills in practice, and so being able to communicate a clear coherent message, with applied real examples, is critical. A cover letter should again be short, sharp and to the point, a page at most. Resist the temptation to go into granular detail about every role and explain every skill you have, instead leave the reader wanting more and so inviting you to interview. As you write, align your experiences with the job description, trying to showcase how your skill set and experiences line up with the requirements of this role. A cover letter should be updated and changed for every application, to ensure that you show how your skills match that particular role on offer. If you find yourself saying, I can't be bothered, then perhaps you are already throwing away your first attempt at a good first impression, and ask yourself if you really are *hardworking* as you stated in your application. Ultimately, your cover letter should outline what you offer to meet the employer's needs, what makes you stand out from the crowd, and how you'll help improve the environment you are going into. Your clarity of message and ability to get your point across succinctly, is key. Leave the short listers wanting more, and you have a greater chance of getting in the room to meet them.

Interview and Task

If you gain an interview, firstly ensure that you reply promptly and professionally to confirm your attendance, whilst if you are unable to make the date proposed, do not be afraid to ask if there is an alternative available. If they really want to interview you, they will accommodate this reasonable request, especially if you are already in another role or have personal commitments. It goes without saying that you should be smart (iron your shirt or blouse!), professional and of course on time. If you are running late for reasons out of your control, make sure that you get in touch to let them know, assuming that it is safe to do so. Before the big day arrives though, it is absolutely pivotal to do your research. That comes in a number of forms, firstly in making sure that you go in with good working knowledge of the organisation you are applying to work for. You can expect to be asked some form of question related to what you know about the organisation, and so it is best to be prepared with some good information. On an individual level, try to see who already works there and where they have been before, recent attainments, aspirations and plans for the future.

You'll likely be asked to undertake some form of task or presentation, either prior to the day, or to present on the day itself. This is a fantastic opportunity to show your practical skills in action, enabling the prospective employers to see your practical skill set. You'll need to use appropriate terminology, language and visuals, alongside presenting back in a manner which excites, that lands the message and would be visually appealing to coaches and players alike. Access to technology might be an issue here, so be innovative, and resourceful in how you approach this, utilising free trials if appropriate, or perhaps asking your network for support and advice in how to complete if required.

Questions asked in an interview will vary from place to place, however you can always expect similar themes. You'll need to be prepared to answer honestly about you and your experiences, bringing your education and practical work to life. Again here, try to link this back towards the role at hand, to show how you fit into the organisation. You'll be asked about culture and team ethos, which are critical to successful organisations, whilst you should also expect to be asked around the use of performance analysis holistically in the environment, what you might do in a difficult scenario, and what some of your biggest work on's still are. There will be hard questions, and there will be some you are less sure on, and so ask for clarification if required and for the question to be framed with an example. At the end of any interview, you'll be asked if you have any questions; this is vital, always have some questions prepared which showcase your initiative, your intrigue and your genuine interest in learning more about the role. An interview is as much an opportunity for you to know more about the job, as it is for the employers to know more about you. And of course, do ask when you might hear back, which is more than a reasonable question, and may help aid any anxieties or concerns of 'should I have heard by now?'.

If the decision goes in your favour, then congratulations! It is a truly exciting time and the start of a fantastic new opportunity for you. Be prepared when you take that call though and have questions ready around salary, working locations and dynamics, alongside potential start dates, bearing in mind any existing notice periods. From there, ensure that you bring your vigour, passion and innovation into the role and truly make the most of it. If it is not the outcome you were hoping for then ensure that you ask for (and insist on) some personal feedback on what you can do to improve. If it is not forthcoming, ask for written or verbal follow up conversations and seek honest feedback, no matter how frustrating it might be to have missed out this time. Be bold, ask to volunteer in the organisation for a week, or shadow perhaps, and finish by thanking them for their time and wishing well for the season ahead.

Exit Routes

Though popular as a career path and a times an exceptionally rewarding role, performance analysis is demanding. The profession demands significant time (almost always antisocial), travel, missed birthdays, Christmases spent away, relinquishment of time with loved ones and difficult decisions. As a result, for many (of course not all) the career span can be short and analysts start to look elsewhere for longer term prospects. Many now look to teaching or lecturing, with a number of ex-analysts with significant practical experience helping drive the applied nature of performance analysis education. This is a significant benefit for those coming through, who learn from analysts who have been (or still are) involved at the highest level. Others will exit into management roles in sport science, moving away from the fire of daily delivery and instead into strategic leadership and planning.

In order to move into any of these roles, thinking ahead whilst still in full-time practical work about constantly enhancing and developing your skill set is vital. This might perhaps be taking on additional roles in the environment, leading on IDT conversations, driving collaboration with Universities or organising and developing school outreach activity. Depending on the future role considered, these will prove valuable in deciphering a new direction and providing a challenging yet strategically informed and objective vision for the next role which is embarked upon.

Concluding Remarks

Though particularly competitive to gain full-time employment, aspiring performance analysts should take heart from the growing number of opportunities to develop their skills. Investing time in the right opportunities with applied experience at the heart is absolutely vital to success as an analyst in the industry. Attention to detail not only in the role, but in the application and interview process is critical, establishing yourself as a serious candidate with exceptional attention to detail for the role at hand, key attributes for an excellent analyst. A humbleness, willingness to continually learn and desire for success throughout, will form a significant part of any aspiring analyst's toolkit.

Reference

Butterworth, A.D., & Turner, D.J. (2014). Becoming a performance analyst: Autoethnographic reflections on and facilitated transformational growth. *Reflective Practice, 15*(5), 552–562.

9

HEALTH, SAFETY AND ETHICS FOR THE PROFESSIONAL PRACTITIONER

Andrew Butterworth and Peter O'Donoghue

Introduction

Health and safety of performance analysts is an important but much overlooked area of performance analysis. O'Donoghue (2014) gave a keynote presentation on health and safety issues in performance analysis at the World Congress of Performance Analysis of Sport X in Opatija, Croatia, in September 2014. This was a useful wake up call to organisations employing performance analysts as well as to practitioners. However, the abstract only exists within the conference proceedings and the slides are not published anywhere for public access. Much of the material is now out of date due to advances in performance analysis hardware and software as well as laws and regulations about using display screen equipment being updated. Within the Routledge Studies in Sports Performance Analysis series of books, health and safety issues in performance analysis practice have only been covered briefly in the ethics chapter of O'Donoghue et al.'s (2018, p. 132) book. This chapter therefore explores materials relating to various health and safety considerations that practitioners should be aware of, including those analysts who are accustomed to long working hours, in poor conditions for low remuneration. This chapter commences with a serious example of a health and safety issue personally experienced by one of the chapter's authors before going on to cover laws and regulations to be complied with by organisations employing performance analysts.

Motivation

In 2013, one of the authors of this chapter, Peter O'Donoghue, blacked out while driving late one night after doing analysis work for a squad. This experience motivated Peter to devote his 2014 keynote address at the World Congress of

DOI: 10.4324/9781003226659-9

Performance Analysis of Sport X to health and safety issues. The presentation was given but was never written up as a full paper, leaving this as a neglected area within sports performance analysis. Now, nine years after the incident, this chapter seeks to give an up-to-date coverage of health and safety issues in the professional practice of performance analysis. Firstly, Peter will briefly describe the incident and the relevant background context.

I was working full time as a university academic and also working as a volunteer analyst for a squad. One of the squad's matches occurred during an important week of the academic year. There were important meetings and classes to attend the day before and the day after the match. This meant that I was unable to travel with the rest of the squad and would not be staying in the hotel with the squad for this match. Instead, I had to drive 2 hours to join the squad at the match venue on match day. At the match venue, I set up my tripod and video camera and was able to find a spare desk to set my computer on. The match started at 8pm and it would be close to 10pm by the time it finished. The position I was video recording the match from was ideal for me to key in most of what the coaches wanted live while the match was being recorded. The filming and live coding of the match went to plan, however there were some additional descriptors that needed to be added during post-match analysis. If I had started the post-match analysis at the venue, I might not have completed this to transfer the information to the coaches before the squad departed for the hotel. Indeed, I might not have been able to complete the post-match analysis before the venue closed its doors for the evening. So I decided to travel to the hotel to complete the post-match analysis there, copy the video and codes onto the coaches' machines and then drive home for work the next day. It was getting close to 11pm by the time my car was exiting the venue and I was on my way to the hotel. I arrived at the hotel, and it was close to midnight when set up my computer at a convenient place to do the post-match analysis. There had been some time lost getting a parking ticket for the hotel car park because I was not a guest. The time after a match can be very busy for the squad. They need to eat, players may need massage therapy and the coaches typically want to touch base with players about critical aspects of the match ahead of the full match analysis being presented. It was around 2am when I finally copied the video and codes onto the coaches' machines. I immediately set off back home, quite content that the squad had the information they needed for the post-match debriefing the next morning. Sometime before then, the coaches would need to select the most important statistics and video sequences to discuss with the players. So it is important to recognise that the coaches were also involved in the analysis, and were also under serious time pressure ahead of the debriefing. I'm not sure whether they stayed up after 2am to select the clips or if this was done the next morning before the debriefing. While I was driving on the motorway, I suddenly found myself to have drifted half way into the next lane. I had blacked out for a second or so. Basically I'd fallen to sleep at the wheel of my car for a short period. I realised with horror what had just happened and eased the car back into the first lane. My immediate thoughts were that I could have had an accident and that I needed to stay awake for the rest of the journey home. Nine years later, I can't recall any yawning or feelings of drowsiness prior to blacking out. I had been focussed on the analysis I was doing earlier in the evening and making what I thought were good decisions to help me complete the post-match analysis. I remember adjusting the heating in the car, I might even have opened the window a little, tried things with radio to make sure I stayed awake for the final part of the journey. I got home ok and slept well before the next day at work. Towards the weekend, I joined the squad for their next match. This time I took the train. I mentioned what had happened to the squad management. They were naturally very concerned.

This account from Peter highlights one health and safety issue, which may have been experienced by some practising performance analysts elsewhere. The issue is volume of work leading to potential fatigue that could lead to other negative consequences depending on the circumstances, which will be discussed later in this chapter. As has already been mentioned, this incident motivated Peter to give a keynote address on health and safety issues in 2014 and to contribute to this chapter. In this chapter, we'll discuss the following health and safety issues from a 'current' and reality perspective, alongside suggestions and improvements that might be made;

- working conditions and remuneration,
- intellectual property right,
- ergonomics and using display screen equipment,
- camera position,
- volume of work,
- health risks,
- vulnerability.

Working Conditions and Remuneration

There are many different types of performance analyst practitioner (Martin et al., 2021), with some described as video coaches, others described as 'scouts', and others having titles like 'Head of Insights'. There has been widespread use of unpaid interns to provide performance analysis services. The most high-profile example of this was a job advert appearing on the UK Sport website that was discussed in *The Independent* newspaper (Taylor, 2013). The advert was for a performance analyst internship at Reading Football Club. It was advertised as a full-time, year-long role, requiring the successful applicant to attend all of the first team's home and away fixtures. The advert stated that the role involved 'unsociable hours', there was no pay, no travelling expenses and that the successful applicant would need to provide their own transport. The successful applicant would need to have experience working as an analyst at least in semi-professional football, be experienced in using video analysis packages that were listed, and would either have to already have a postgraduate qualification or be on their way to achieving this. The article discussed one view that interns doing real work are entitled to the minimum wage. This may be the case in the UK, but people have done voluntary work in many fields and so the use of unpaid volunteer analysts is not likely to be illegal. During the article in *The Independent*, Reading Football Club responded that internships are a great opportunity for aspiring football analysts, that such internships attract a large number of applicants, and that a number of interns have progressed to becoming full-time professional analysts. Indeed, Reading has a history of employing professional performance analysts.

Sometimes, we can see organisations trying to justify the use of unpaid interns and volunteers by devaluing the work they do. A particularly annoying example of this is the use of the term 'coding monkeys', referring to the manual logging of events which often falls to interns. The fact is that performance analysis needs data and not all data can be gathered automatically. Without reliable data being gathered, there is no data analysis or analytics work that can be done. There is no profiling, no trend analysis and no data science insights. Thus, dismissing those who gather sports performance data as 'coding monkeys' is at best an ignorant point of view.

There are some sports with very limited budgets for any kind of sports science support. They would like to have performance analysis support for their athletes but they want it on a 'shoestring' budget. Analysts can find themselves wishing to promote performance analysis by volunteering to be an analyst with such a sport, and not wishing to undervalue the profession. Such sports need to be encouraged to seek sponsorship to support performance analysis services or use other means to provide financial support. Analysts who already have paid roles should be discouraged from working as volunteers if this simply delays a sport from creating a paid analysis position for graduates seeking careers in this area.

Another area of potential concern is the use of unpaid placement students to provide performance analysis services to national governing bodies and sports clubs. Universities certainly want their students to undertake relevant work experience because it enhances the employability of graduates. Students typically need to do something for a work experience module or placement year, and being able to include experience with a professional sports organisation on their CV is certainly beneficial. The sports organisation can also provide references for students who have worked with them when they are applying for paid roles later on. So at first glance, the links between universities and sports organisations seem mutually beneficial, and in most cases they are. There are undesirable practices, however, that we would not wish to see when it comes to the use of work experience students to provide performance analysis services. For example, an organisation could use new work experience students each year, never creating a full-time analyst role. Other examples of concerning practice are where organisations require work experience students to do an excessive number of hours, far exceeding the number of hours required by their work experience module. A 20 UK credit point module requires 200 effort hours, 80 hours of which would be direct placement work. The main issue with students exceeding this is that the additional work may be at the expense of marks in other modules on their programme of study leading towards an imbalance of focus.

A key challenge for university programmes with work-experience modules will be to ensure that the industry does not become over-reliant on unpaid placement students and interns. There are now numerous UK universities offering masters programmes in sports performance analysis, so there are plenty of students wanting to work with professional organisations as part of their masters programmes. Where large numbers of unpaid placement students contribute to the industry, it can block the creation of good well-paid performance analysis jobs. That said, there are now a number of organisations who have responded positively, providing a good working remuneration for the hours completed on placements or interns, in addition to other benefits in kind.

Intellectual Property Rights

When considering the rights of employees in the sports performance analysis industry, it is also important to consider the rights of employers. Professional performance analysts are typically employees of organisations, although there are some freelance performance analysts who provide services to client organisations on a consultancy basis. Analysts employed by clubs and sports governing bodies typically work with equipment belonging to those organisations as well as with data largely owned by those organisations. There may be some data used by organisations and their analysts that comes from third-party providers and used within the terms of contracts agreed by the organisations and the third party providers. When analysts move from one job to another, they should not be taking data owned by their previous employer with them. This applies to data collected by the analyst and their former colleagues in the organisation as well as data from third party providers.

Similarly, when interns or work-experience students are working as performance analysts with professional organisations, they should not be taking intellectual property belonging to the organisation away from the organisation without permission. Agreements should be made up-front about what kinds of material can be included in portfolios and presentations for assessment purposes. It is undesirable for interns and work-experience students to be taking intellectual property away from the organisation without permission. It is also undesirable for work-experience students to be working on courseworks, expecting to be able to use examples, to be told this is not permitted after they have already done most of the placement hours they have been set.

Although this chapter is about performance analysis in practice rather than academic research into sports performance analysis, there are occasions where the two overlap. For example, a practising performance analyst might be doing a master's programme and using their analysis role as a source of material for a work-experience module and/or a dissertation. There are potential ethical issues here about disclosure of how performance analysis is used by the squad. Some practices may give the squad an edge and they might not want details of these practices shared within a thesis or coursework report that could find its way into the hands of rival clubs. The analyst should seek permission from the squad to use the experience of being a squad analyst in their academic work. They should be clear about university regulations about courseworks being visible to supervising lecturers, staff involved in moderation and external examiners. The analyst and the club should agree on the things that can be disclosed within university courseworks and those things that must not be.

Ergonomics and Using Display Screen Equipment

Ergonomics is concerned with the interaction between people and equipment when tasks are being performed in the work environment (HSE, nodate). Ergonomics is sometimes referred to as human factors engineering and is a massive area of research in transport, assembly line work and office working environments. Ergonomics seeks to ensure tasks can be fulfilled minimising the risk of repetitive strain injury and industrial accidents. A simple example of an ergonomics development was attaching wheels to bins and luggage to make them easier to move. With respect to performance analysis, ergonomics is relevant to using video recording equipment as well as computers and peripheral devices. Consider something like the Hi-Pod system used to allow elevated views of performance (HIPOD, nodate). This is quite bulky equipment that needs to be transported to venues where performances are being filmed. Therefore, ergonomics needs to consider not just the use of the equipment but also how it is packaged, transported and set up. Peter O'Donoghue, in contributing to this chapter, considers his working environment:

> As I was working on different sections of this chapter, it did occur to me that my working environment might not be ideal. During the 2020 and 2021 lockdowns, I was working at home and preferred to work standing up, especially when the gym was closed. I set my laptop computer on top of some box files on a kitchen work surface so it would be at a comfortable height for me to operate the keyboard and view the screen. In truth, this probably was not ideal. To be fair to my employer at the time, they offered to provide me with an adjustable standing desk for use in my home. I declined this offer because I felt my house was cluttered enough and it was difficult to dispose of some items in my house that I wanted to recycle during the lockdowns. This raises a point about analyst responsibility. There may be occasions where employers have fulfilled their obligations but analysts have continued to work in unauthorised ways without complying with health and safety instructions or guidance from employers. Given the nature of work in sports performance analysis, analysts do need to prioritise their own health and safety, no matter how keen they are to make progress with tasks.

The UK's Health and Safety Executive have specified employers' obligations to workers who use display screen equipment continuously for an hour or more as part of their daily jobs (HSE, 2022a). The Health and Safety (Display Screen Equipment) Regulations of 1992 apply together with amendments made in 2002. Display screen equipment includes PCs, laptop computers, tablets and smartphones. The regulations apply whether working in an office, at home, or at multiple venues. They apply whether items of equipment are on fixed desks or if 'hot desks' are being used. The regulations do not apply where workers use display screen equipment for short periods or infrequently. The use of display screen equipment by performance analysts depends on the sport, the information required by coaches and players, the depth of analysis and the number of analysts contributing to the work. In most cases, performance analysts are required to use display screen equipment for prolonged periods. Therefore, performance analysis work falls within the law relating to using display screen equipment.

The risks involved in incorrect use of display screen equipment include fatigue, eye strain as well as pains in the neck, shoulders, back, arms, wrists and hands (HSE, 2022a). Employers are legally obliged to carry out risk assessments where workers use display screen equipment on a daily basis continuously for an hour or more. Where risks are identified, steps must be taken to reduce these. The Health and Safety Executive's description of risk assessment is where a 'workstation' is being used. However, the regulations apply where any display screen equipment are being used. It is, therefore, necessary for employers to assess the specific risks associated with using display screen equipment within their workers' roles. This needs to consider the type of display screen equipment, the tasks requiring display screen equipment to be used, working conditions, furniture and environment within which work is being carried out. The risk assessment should also consider any relevant disabilities of workers and any other special requirements they may have. Sports performance analysis roles have some unique risks, as many other job types do. The usability of video analysis software for the given task should be considered before committing to a particular piece of software. The system should be tailored for use in the given sport in a way that best supports data gathering and analysis tasks. In some situations, matches need to be filmed using camera equipment connected to computer equipment. In some situations, the camera may be fixed during data recording, but in other situations it may be necessary to zoom and pan during filming. Organisations should consider whether a separate camera operator is needed in such situations to help minimise risks. The benefits of employing an additional camera operator include that operating a single piece of equipment (such as a laptop computer) is easier to do in an ergonomic manner than if an analyst is simultaneously operating a camera as well. Analysts will also find themselves expected (or needing) to work in many different places including at poorly designed hotel desks, on coach or plane journeys (Figure 9.1), balancing laptops on laps and in temporary worktop settings.

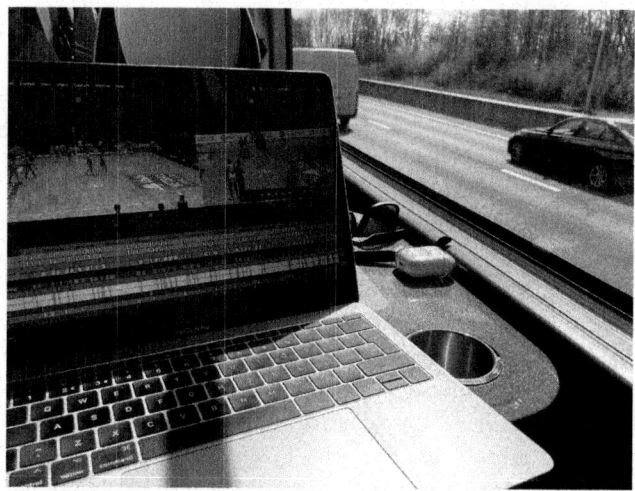

FIGURE 9.1 Working condition on coach travel.

Organisations employing performance analysts, whether professionally or on a voluntary basis, are encouraged to use the Health and Safety Executive's checklist for working with display screen equipment (HSE, 2022b). This identifies the regulations that need to be complied with and provides a table allowing various aspects of using keyboards, mouse devices, display screens within the working environment to be checked or noted as areas requiring further action. Examples are given of ergonomically risky ways of working with equipment as well as safer arrangements. The checklist not only covers hardware and the physical environment where hardware is used, but also covers the readability of what is displayed on screens by the software systems being used within roles. There are some aspects that are not covered in the checklist, which the checklist alerts users to. These include the need for training to use equipment and taking breaks during tasks. These should also be addressed within wider risk management processes.

Health and safety training for workers using display screen equipment is required by law in the UK and is a responsibility of employers (HSE, 2022a). The training should be about risks involved in using display screen equipment and how to avoid or minimise these. It should also cover the working environment, furniture and posture, whilst also considering adjustments to display screens to avoid reflections and glare. Taking breaks and changes of activity must also be covered within training, which should familiarise workers with how to raise health and safety concerns and risk assessment processes should be included.

Prolonged use of display screen equipment risks temporary short sightedness and headaches. Analysts should ensure the screen is well positioned for their task, ensure lighting conditions are as suitable as possible for working with display screens and take regular breaks. UK law requires employers to pay for eye tests for workers who use display screen equipment on a daily basis continually for an hour or more if they ask for one. This should be a full eye test conducted by an optometrist or doctor, including a vision test and eye examination. The eye test may reveal that workers need specialist glasses to do their job. Employers should provide glasses where workers require them exclusively for working with display screen equipment.

In the UK, employers are required by law to plan breaks or changes of activity for workers who use display screen equipment (HSE, 2022a). This is especially important where there are no natural breaks within working routines to take phone calls, etc. These breaks should allow users to get up, if they are seated, stretch, change posture and move around. The frequency and duration of breaks has not been specified within the regulations. It is recognised that the frequency and duration of breaks depend on the nature of the work being done. Display screen users should take frequent shorter breaks rather than long breaks more infrequently. Ideally, display screen users should be able to choose when to take breaks. This is possible with lapse-time analysis where previously recorded sports performances are being analysed. However, where live coding is necessary, it might be impossible for analysts to take a break from display screen use during a match period. The Health and Safety Executive guidance mentions software that monitors computer use and reminds users to take regular breaks (HSE, 2022a).

Camera Position

Many analysts do not need to video record matches themselves. Some are given access to video feeds at match venues, others use existing video repositories, while some others analyse performance without the need for video at all. A recent development has been the use of IP cameras from within a performance analysis laboratory or other designated space. These cameras can be controlled manually with a joystick allowing zooming and panning to follow the action, or automatically with advanced artificial intelligence and algorithms. Essentially, the analyst benefits from an elevated viewing position without personally having to work at height. This chapter section is concerned with analysts who need to film matches themselves as part of their analysis process.

The most important factor in choosing a location to film from is the quality of the video images to be provided as feedback to players and coaches. In game sports as well as racket sports, the best viewing position is an elevated view often from behind one end of the playing surface rather than a side on view. However, it is not always possible to set up the video camera from an elevated position behind the playing area. For example, the venue may have elevated viewing positions within stands at the sides of the playing area but there may not actually be stands at the ends of the playing area and it might not be possible to set up a platform behind the playing area. In some venues, where filming can be done from behind the playing area, the view might be restricted. For example, it might not be possible to see players' feet when they are at the near end of the playing area.

This is especially true where the playing surface is several feet below the first row of spectator seating.

When filming at any venue, the analyst needs to comply with all health and safety regulations of the venue. Some venues will insist on Portable Appliance Testing (PAT) equipment being brought into the venue. Analysts may also have to provide details of what they are filming and what the images are being used for. This is sometimes for child protection purposes, and analysts are typically given a badge to wear as well as a sticker for their equipment to signify that they have registered to film at the venue. In recent years, there has been a noticeable breakdown in the enforcement of these regulations. Friends and relatives of players often film performances with mobile devices without having considered that they may be breaking the child protection regulations of the venue. This may all seem innocent enough, but there is always the possibility that someone unconnected with the players may be filming without permission. The use of mobile phones is now so common place that some tournaments don't place restrictions on their use. For example, the terms and conditions of tickets for the Women's UEFA Euro 2022 tournament prohibits video cameras and professional cameras. This is very different to the terms and conditions stated on tickets for professional soccer matches in the English Football League before 2010 (O'Donoghue, 2010, p. 118). Specifically, the terms and conditions of a Cardiff City Football Club ticket in the 2008–2009 season included

> No person may bring into the ground any equipment which is capable of recording or transmitting audio or visual material or any information or data relating to any match, or the ground. Mobile phones are permitted for personal use only.

The feasibility of using any viewing position may also depend on access to a power supply. It is not always possible to set up video recording equipment safely from a given viewing position as the equipment and personnel operating it may be blocking spectator entrance and exit routes. Any cables used with the video recording equipment need to be taped down to minimise the risk of people tripping over them. Equally there may be a need for tables to place laptops or other equipment on, which may also limit the space from which filming can occur, since these inevitably take up space which might stop certain tickets from being sold and a subsequent loss of income.

There are still occasions where analysts film matches from risky positions. One of this chapter's authors, Peter O'Donoghue, recalls having to film in a sports hall where the only elevated position was a platform 20–30 feet up a ladder at the back of the sports hall. The platform had railings around it and the ladder had a safety cage around it. Peter had to make two separate trips up the ladder to bring his tripod and camera up on the first trip and his computer up on the second trip. It was so high up, that the coach did not see up on the platform at the top of the ladder when first arriving and asked a few of the players if Peter

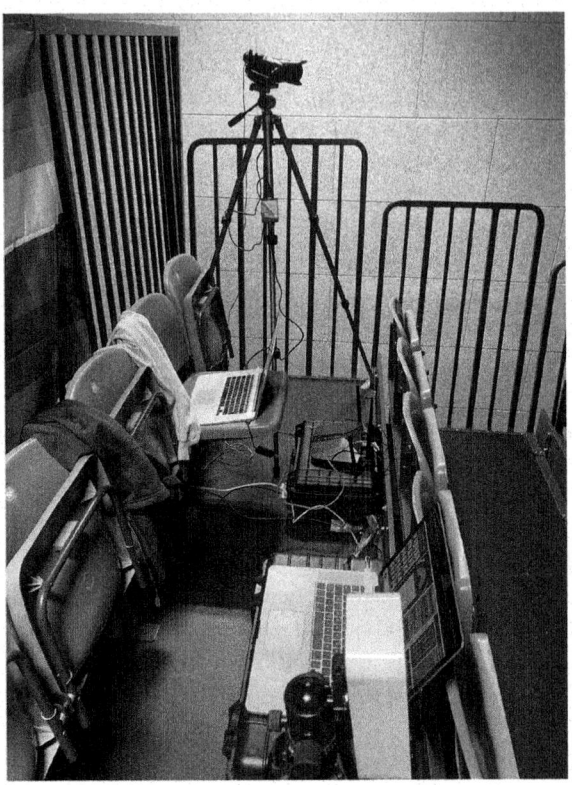

FIGURE 9.2 Temporary stand analysis set up.

was about! The other author of this chapter, Andrew Butterworth, has filmed at the same venue and chose not to ascend the ladder but instead arranged for a platform to be brought in for him to film from. Andrew has also experienced some far from ideal positions at other venues too, including multiple times where it is expected to set up at the back of temporary stands without any access to safe power supplies, tables or chairs. Instead, in these scenarios little thought (if any) is given to the health and safety of the analysts and instead it is just expected that they will work in the very small space confines, as seen in Figure 9.2.

Most venue staff rightly insist on analysts complying with health and safety requirements when filming. We can recall one occasion where an analyst asked for access to an ideal viewing position on a ledge 2.5–3 m off the ground above an entrance door. The venue staff refused to allow this unless the analyst wore a harness. The coach tried to persuade the venue staff to change their decision, but the venue staff quite rightly prioritised health and safety over the quality of footage. The insurance policies held by venues are typically on condition that there are health and safety guidance, procedures and risk assessments. Any violation of such policies and procedures could result in the insurance policy being invalidated.

Volume of Work

There are laws about the number of hours of work that employees do per week. The European Union's Working Time Directive stipulates that employers cannot force employees to work more than 48 hours per week on average including overtime in a 4 month or 17 week period (EU, 2003). This regulation has also been retained by Britain post-BREXIT (UK Government, no date), though employees can work a longer average week than 48 hours by 'opting out' of the 48-hour rule. Employers can ask employees to opt out but cannot force them to do so or dismiss or harm employees if they choose not to opt out. Where employees have opted out of the 48-hour limit, it is advised that an opt out agreement is made between employee and employer. Some classes of worker cannot opt out, for example workers in the transport industry cannot choose to do a longer average working week than 48 hours. In considering whether practising performance analysts should be exceeding 48 hours work per week, it is worth considering other professions where people may be required to exceed the 48-hour average. These include armed forces personnel, emergency service workers, seafarers and sea-fishermen. Managing executives who's work might not be measured on a time basis and who are in control of their own decisions may also find themselves doing more than 48 hours per week on average. A performance analyst working with a squad that competes once per week should be able to complete their weekly data gathering, analysis and briefing-related tasks well within 48 hours. Indeed they should be able to complete this work within 40 hours meaning overtime should not need to be paid. However, the volume of work depends on the detail of analysis required, the ability to live-code matches, the number of squads the analyst is working with and whether individual player analysis is being done as well as team level analysis. It is, therefore, very important that an understanding of the work is established with clear estimates of how long is required to gather data and apply each stage of processing.

The sports organisation needs to consider the value of the information they require and the resources needed for the depth of analysis involved. It may be that they have limited resources to pay for performance analysis services and, therefore, need to be selective about the most important analyses that are required for decision support. It is also important for performance analysts to communicate workload estimates to the organisations they work for. Needs analysis, service planning and reaching service level agreements are components of applied performance analysis practice (Martin et al., 2021). Martin et al. (2021) also recommended the use of service reviews and evaluations. Organisations may simply not realise the amount of work required to produce statistical feedback and telestrated video sequences. There may be an attitude that 'the performance analyst just does that', where squad management believe that a particular outcome of analysis can be produced in a straightforward manner, requiring little time.

Other relevant aspects of the Working Time Directive are that under 18s cannot work more than 8 hours per day or 40 hours per week. There must be

11 consecutive hours of rest from work per day and 24 hours uninterrupted rest from work at least once per week. The reference period for these constraints is 2 weeks. Where employees are required to work more than 6 hours in a day, breaks must be given to employees. Employees are also entitled to at least four weeks paid holiday per year. Employees may also count as night workers if at least three hours of their work shift occurs between midnight and 5 am. The implications of this include that night workers cannot work more than 8 hours per 24-hour period, and are entitled to health assessments before they commence night work.

So far we have concentrated on the EU's Working Time Directive. The US Department of Labor website (no date) specifies federal regulations for the Federal minimum wage, overtime and record keeping. Any work done above a 40-hour working week is counted as overtime and should be paid at least 1.5 times the rate of normal working hours. Employers are responsible for maintaining records of paid work done by employees and payments made to them. In addition to Federal employment laws, there may be additional state laws that employers and employees need to comply with.

Returning to the incident of Peter O'Donoghue falling asleep for a moment when driving back from doing analysis work, it is worth considering this incident in the light of the EU's Working Time Directive. The first thing to mention is that O'Donoghue was working as a volunteer on top of a full-time job. This complicates the situation because voluntary work may not come under the directive. O'Donoghue was not instructed to do this voluntary work by his university employers. Therefore, it is most likely that if he had been killed falling asleep at the wheel of his car, an inquest would not have placed responsibility on anyone else. Remember from O'Donoghue's account that he does not recall experiencing any warning signs of drowsiness or yawning before the incident, and that he did not make the squad management aware of what had happened until afterwards. It is, therefore, important that analysts reading this book understand their responsibilities to themselves and their families. They need to consider the work they are taking on, even if this is voluntary work, and consider the health and safety risks involved. The incident did not necessarily involve any breaches of regulations, and there was not enough analysis work done after midnight for this to qualify as night work. None-the-less, the timing of the work and the need to travel back from the venue in the early hours of the morning presented a risk that O'Donoghue did not manage satisfactorily. It is important that analysts develop relationships within squads that allow them to raise any health and safety concerns. Building relationships is one of five areas of expertise underpinning professional practice in sports performance analysis (Martin et al., 2021) and something considered elsewhere at multiple times in this book.

The quality of analysis work also has an impact on the time required to complete the work. An initial unchecked analysis can produce results in good time for coaches and players to use them to support decisions. However, if the extra time is not taken to perform consistency and completeness checks on the data, reduced data quality can compromise the use of information within the coaching cycle. Some players may question video sequences and might correctly point to examples of miscoded outcomes that reflect negatively upon their performances. This in turn may lead to a mistrust in coaching advice that is supported by the analysis. Analysts themselves may be blamed for lack of attention to detail. However, it needs to be recognised that the quality of work is impacted upon by the resources made available, the amount of work to be done, and how quickly squads need analysis tasks to be turned around.

Health Risks

Some health risks due to sleep deprivation, long working hours, eye strain, poor ergonomics and risky camera positions have already been mentioned in this chapter. There are other more general risks associated with the sedentary nature of some performance analysis tasks. Analysts may be sitting, working on computers, for long periods of time. This is sedentary behaviour that can be associated with risk of cardiovascular disease, diabetes and some cancers (Mayor, 2015). Analysts' diets may also be irregular and of low quality. For example, analysts may find themselves not taking proper meals and eating food from vending machines while continuing to do analysis work. The responsibility of this is largely upon the analyst themselves, but some employers also opt to take on ownership of this, including arranging staff team activities and wellbeing alongside providing food on site for consumption.

Vulnerability

Vulnerability experienced by some performance analysts is relevant to this chapter but has been covered more fully in other chapters of this book. Therefore, we will mention it briefly in this chapter to make the point that is relevant to health and safety at work. Huggan et al. (2014) investigated the experience of an early career performance analyst, finding that they did feel vulnerable and needed to develop in order to act micro-politically to help protect their career and advancement. In this chapter, we are specifically interested in vulnerability, as presented by Huggan et al. (2014), rather than developing micro-political literacy. They acknowledged that previous research has found vulnerabilities due to ideology and the goals of others exist in many work domains. They used a story-telling approach whereby an analyst was interviewed on four occasions about the first ten years of their career as a performance analyst. The storytelling approach has many advantages, for example protecting the identity of the analyst, and being able to integrate theory within the interpretations of the data gathered.

The narrative describes how the analyst perceived the need to sell one's self to decision makers who had the power to use performance analysis within the club or not. Huggan et al. (2014) discussed the vulnerability felt by the analyst when coaching staff were not interested in performance analysis, describing it as 'a battle he could not win in the long term'. They can feel marginalised and that their contribution is not valued. The lack of support may also involve lack of investment in technology needed for the analyst to do their job well. Where there are frequent changes in coaching staff, analysts can feel themselves being 'back at square one' and needing to justify their work again.

Even where the analyst has full support from the coaches and has key 'allies' in other areas of sports science support, there may still be vulnerability where players perceive the analyst as a 'spy' for the coaches. Another area of vulnerability is where analysts feel the need to take on additional work to make them essential to the club. A positive situation discussed in Huggan et al.'s (2014) paper was where an analyst had the support of the club chairperson and was encouraged to speak to them about any difficulties faced working with coaches.

Concluding Remarks

This chapter has covered important health and safety issues in applied performance analysis. Sports performance analysis is a profession, and many performance analysts working in the industry are highly qualified, some at masters level or above. It is important not to undersell the profession, but this chapter has revealed some situations where analysts may be volunteers and interns. Such positions can be useful in gaining work experience, and have led to analysts finding full-time paid positions. However, there is also a danger of the industry becoming over-reliant on unpaid interns and work placement students, and this could block the creation of paid roles for analysts. Analysts can feel vulnerable where their work is not valued or coaches and players don't buy into performance analysis. Clearly, an organisation cannot be forced to use performance analysis if it does not wish to. Therefore, more research work is needed to demonstrate the effectiveness of performance analysis based feedback. This is an important area of research that is underdeveloped compared with descriptive studies of sports performance. This book is a useful source of material, much of it original research, that can help stimulate further research in this area.

Performance analysts can find themselves working long hours and this can lead to serious risks as has been described in this chapter. Poor diet, irregular eating patterns and lack of exercise can all be detrimental to the health of analysts. Sleep deprivation must also be avoided, especially where the analyst may be driving after long hours of analysis work. Analysts need to raise concerns about such issues with the organisations they work for, because these organisations may have no idea of the issues otherwise. This chapter has also covered health and safety risks in applied performance analysis that come from the use of equipment in the work environment. There are regulations relating to the use of display screens at work that must be complied with. The camera positions used by analysts should also be chosen ensuring that venue policies and procedures are followed and that the risk of accidents is minimised.

References

EU (2003). *Directive 2003/88/EC of the European Parliament and of the Council of 4 November 2003 concerning certain aspects of the organisation of working time.* Retrieved 8th July 2022 from: https://eur-lex.europa.eu/legal-content/EN/TXT/?uri=CELEX %3A32003L0088&qid=1670618121872.

HIPOD (no date). *Hi-Pod: elevate your game.* Retrieved 7th July 2022 from: https://www.hipod.com/.

HSE (2022a). *Working safely with display screen equipment.* Retrieved 11th June 2022 from: https://www.hse.gov.uk/msd/dse/.

HSE (2022b). *Display screen equipment (DSE) workstation checklist.* Retrieved 11th June 2022 from: https://www.hse.gov.uk/pubns/ck1.pdf.

HSE (n.d.). *Ergonomics and human factors at work.* Retrieved 7th July 2022 from: https://www.hse.gov.uk/pubns/indg90.pdf.

Huggan, R., Nelson, L., & Potrac, P. (2014). Developing micropolitical literacy in professional soccer: a performance analyst's tale. *Qualitative Research in Sport Exercise and Health, 7*(4), 504–520.

Martin, D., O'Donoghue, P.G., Bradley, J., & McGrath, D. (2021). Developing a framework for professional practice in applied performance analysis. *International Journal of Performance Analysis in Sport, 21*(6), 845–888.

Mayor, S. (2015). Stand during working day to prevent health risks of sedentary jobs, says guidance. *BMJ, 2015,* 350.

O'Donoghue, P.G. (2010). *Research methods for sports performance analysis.* London: Routledge.

O'Donoghue, P.G. (2014). *Health and safety issues in performance analysis.* Keynote address at the World Congress of Performance Analysis in Sport X, Opatija, Croatia.

O'Donoghue, P.G., Holmes, L., & Robinson, G. (2018). *Doing a research project in sports performance analysis.* London: Routledge.

Taylor, J. (2013), Unpaid, bad hours, and you have to watch Reading: Is the is the worst job in football? *The Independent.* Retrieved 4th July 2022 from: https://www.independent.co.uk/sport/football/news/unpaid-bad-hours-and-you-have-to-watch-reading-is-this-the-worst-job-in-football-8569387.html.

UK Government (n.d.). *Maximum weekly working hours.* Retrieved 8th July 2022 from: https://www.gov.uk/maximum-weekly-working-hours.

US Department of Labor (n.d.). *Working hours.* Retrieved 8th July 2022 from: https://www.dol.gov/general/topic/workhours.

10

ECONOMIC ISSUES AND SOLUTIONS IN PERFORMANCE ANALYSIS

Andrew Butterworth

Introduction

Elite high-end performance analysis workflows typically demand expensive hardware and software to be fully functional. With the cost of hardware continuing to grow, coupled with booming software contracts and add ons, the economics of performance analysis provision can spiral. Whilst for economically strong sports this is not an obstacle, but for those with more budget constraints and those unable to invest at all, it provides a considerable block to progressing performance analysis workflows. Having established some of the contemporary and innovative technologies emerging in the field earlier in this book, this chapter will first consider the growing use of these technologies in day-to-day workflows and some associated costs. Useful for current analysts with less budget and also those aspiring to gain positions, this chapter explores the restricting problems with expensive technologies in performance analysis, whilst also offering practical hands on advice for cheaper or free alternatives with applied examples to assist.

Problems: Keeping Pace

The evolutionary drive and increasing use of computers in sports performance analysis is twofold, from innovators and expert practitioners keen to grow efficiency and stimulate further performance enhancements for their athletes, coupled with a parallel growth in digital technologies. Together these empower speedier feedback and enhanced decision making in the moment as sporting pursuits evolve. Whilst exciting and offering up opportunity for genuine innovation and practice enhancement, the growth also brings about challenges and sometimes significant cost implications.

DOI: 10.4324/9781003226659-10

Such is the growth of performance analysis technologies in just a short few years, the workflows and tools of high-end elite performance analysis departments are near unrecognisable from just a few years previous. Gone are the days of manual messaging and landline phones to communicate to pitch side, in are the days of wireless communication, automated artificial intelligence (AI)-enabled filming and near instant video replays for coaches. For some sports the change was slower to adopt, not necessarily for lacking of want or trying, but because of restrictive governing body or league arrangements. For example, in English football the league restrictions did not allow for any technology on benches until very recently, where you'll now be hard pressed to watch any match or highlights without seeing coaches engaged with their tablet devices on the bench or with wireless headphones in linked back to the analysts. Meanwhile in elite netball, on the international stage when early innovators adopted technology on their benches, the international federation soon blocked the use, citing unfair advantage.

Culture and willingness to engage have also impacted uptake too, with elite rugby coaches having adopted technology into their match day workflows many years prior, and analysis intervention in the moment forming a critical part of coach decision making. It is rare, if ever, to see a rugby coach pitch-side delivering information, with nearly all instead opting for a bird's eye perspective alongside their trusted analysts, digesting vital performance analysis data to help make decisions. Many other sports adopt these workflows too, with elite netball (since the federation relaxed its stance) being one such which has started to engage heavily with innovative and pioneering coaches engaging with different technologies and analysis methodologies, seeking to advance practice. In football, the cultural adaptation took longer and still evolves today with some managers historically having sat with analysts, such as Nigel Pearson during his second stint at Leicester City, who forced initially through a touchline ban, discussed and ingested performance analysis data, opting to stay beyond the lengths of the ban given the benefits it bought. Media coverage at the time bought headlines questioning this practice though, and he soon returned to the touchline. Engagement in football today largely revolves around radio contact back to an analyst and mobile technologies on the bench.

Enabling any of these methodologies can start to become prohibitive though, and soon costs start to grow, primarily when concerning the technology itself with multiple component parts required to run a fully immersive and technologically discipline. Costs spiral further with the human resource required to operate such departments with multiple analysts often required in order to enact the full wishes of the coach, meaning investment in personnel and then ongoing professional development and upskilling for them too. With many now seeing the use of performance analysis and technology as a core part of the evolving coaching process, keeping abreast of the latest developments and implementing them in practice can become desirable but unattainable to some given the financial strain. The problem is not really new though, and since performance analysis is culturally embedded as a technologically rich discipline, it has in turn has been prohibitive for many.

The Cult of Mac

Since the popularity of performance analysis grew as a sports science discipline, it has always leant closely towards evolving powerful hardware and in particular Apple products. Stop an elite sport analyst on a match day and check their bags, and more often than not you'll find half an Apple store contained within their Peli cases. Such has been the dominance of the technology giant, analysts now predominantly rely on each of the hardware options with multiple MacBooks, iPads, iPhones, Apple TVs, Apple AirPorts and Airpods to indicate just a few of the technologies used on most typical set up's, not to mention the multitude of adaptors. Lessons are learned here very quickly for a player or coach to never be behind the analysts in the security bag check queue at the airport or entering to a venue!

Lessons too are perhaps needed in the *necessity* of continually updating what is in the bags, with promises made of even more power, speed and processing capabilities in the latest releases. Often accompanied with flashy launches, Apple products promise better capabilities and supremacy than the last, whilst annoyingly changing the ports and connectors meaning more adaptors are required to be purchased. For instance, the removal of traditional USB, SD slot and HDMI connectors from previous machines opting instead for USB-C only (meaning more adaptors!), before reverting that decision in the latest release. In addition, M1 chips, retina displays and longer lasting batteries have all come into production too, which given the frequency of updates make it hard to understand what really is the latest and most efficient hardware required.

Research in football suggests that 88% of analysts use Apple-based products for their analysis workflows (Wright *et al.,* 2013), cementing the dominance of a powerful yet expensive provision. Whilst firm research isn't yet available to confirm this percentage in other sports, we need not look further than the gantry of most sport events, to know which machines and powers are being harnessed most frequently. There are viable PC-based options too, though that said, software that have until now been exclusively PC based (e.g. NacSport) have recently launched Mac versions, signalling a further nod to the continued dominance of Apple products for hardware in analysis.

Software Compatibility and Subscriptions

Further complications, and sometimes costs, come when considering the compatibility of software with these latest machines also. As new hardware models are released, the major software companies need significant time to perform appropriate testing to ensure smooth running. In the past, analysts have been all too keen to upgrade their MacBooks to the latest OS X and slightly enhanced aesthetics, only to discover dropped video frames, or worse still incompatibility with capture conversion devices leading to crashing software or no picture at all. For the analyst, this means frustration, closing constant pop-up messages about upgrading and patience, all whilst waiting for the new specialist software versions to come to fruition and confirmation of their successful operating on the new OS.

The bigger, expensive, problematic and more recent problem comes in the shape of a shift away from one-off capital expenditure costs for investment in software licences, to annual renewal subscriptions. Whereas in the past a licence would be purchased per machine for life, perhaps with a nominal annual maintenance fee or more reasonable upgrade offers, virtually all of the major technology companies have shifted solely to annual costs. This means that year on year, to maintain service levels provided another renewal must be negotiated (usually at a higher price), or be pressed towards initial multi-year deals of four years+ at the risk that the software becomes overtaken by a competitor in that time. It is reported that some elite football clubs software bills to single companies come in at close to £200,000 per year and whilst that might *only* be a week's wages for the third choice goalkeeper in some clubs, even for the richest organisations justifying and sustaining these annual costs on top of hardware is simply unviable for most. Depending on the provider and deal struck, that figure might not even include data access, telestration or collaboration tools either, which come at an additional premium. It is important to note that not all companies adopt this aggressive sales tactic, with many more flexible and accommodating and some even still offering single purchase one off fees, though these are increasingly rare. Given the brand-loyalty to certain companies for some, reputation, reluctance to change or unwillingness to re-train an entire department, loyalty in performance analysis software often come at a price.

Additional Hardware

Of course, none of the above is relevant unless video is first ingested into the machines before being loaded onto an analysis software or two. As established in Chapter 2, there are now a plethora of hardware options for recording video footage, some with AI-enabled automation and some still the traditional tripod and manually pan approach. The cost of a full-automated system to cover multiple pitches at a training ground and multiple angles in a stadium runs quickly into tens of thousands. In many environments now, there is a desire to have near instant access to video replay and data on the side-line. This too comes at a cost with the need firstly for network infrastructure which for fixed home venues would hopefully be wired to ensure connectivity, though that may not be possible depending on the filming vantage point, or for a portable away game solution, wireless transmission devices such as Ruckus access points. Couple this with a state-of-the-art iPad, and yet another different software licence to mount on that iPad, and monies are once again significantly piling up. In the changing rooms at quarter or half time, there might be the desire to watch some footage back to help players visually see the game, whilst there are many solutions for this, it is typically going to involve another hardware device and more software, not to mention the HD screen or projector.

Human Resource

Within the evolving AI and algorithm-driven age, there is almost an assumption that this is the direction of travel for the *best* analysis environments. There is much to be said for automation and it has indeed made huge strides forward in assisting our processes, saved considerable time and made workflows more efficient. However, even with that there remains a need for humans to be part of the process in helping collect, analyse and crucially deliver information back to end users. Even where automated filming is becoming more prevalent for video collection, there are issues with reliability, algorithm accuracy and framing play appropriately. And while AI-driven coding is beginning coming to the fore too, we are still a considerable way off fully automated coding which can accurately take in all events of a dynamic sport and reliably code them in a consistent manner. Even as reliability does improve, we'd likely still have questions about the trust in a system, not to mention the near impossible task of asking an algorithm to be inside a coach or analysts mind and code philosophy-based passages of play which often defy accurate or fully informed definition. There is also the problem of data quantity, with the volume and range of metrics being produced larger than ever and needing extensive management and interpretation to become useful for practice. When then delivering back whilst automated reports and telestration help considerably with time to produce reports, as the ultimate recipients of an analysts work, athletes are not robots, nor should they be treated like them with non-interactive reporting, just because expensive technologies allow for more automation.

There is and will remain the need for significant investment into human resources to operate a performance analysis department. Even if automation in some processes is enabled, athletes and coaches alike still crave human interaction and insight into the delivery of their analysis work. To that end, organisations will also need to consider the cost of investing in humans to deliver this with costs needing to include salaries, pensions, insurances, medical, travel, food and many other aspects too. As discovered earlier in this book, the industry remains largely underpaid for full-time roles, and whilst thankfully unpaid internships are now more rare, starting salaries for entry-level analysis roles barely make it above low twenties, which in comparison to some football player wages seems somewhat out of kilter, though needless to say that debate will not be opened here. That is not the case everywhere, and some are rewarded much better for their work, especially since they've likely spent tens of thousands in tuition, courses and 'accreditations' to get to that point. Even so, the costs will still mount relatively quickly for analysis personnel, especially if the roll out of analysis is to filter through to age group and academy set ups. Therefore, the cost of human resource to turn the department will also have to be considered, built in next to the technological costs and wider budgetary needs of the organisation.

All of these technologies come at a cost if the top-end offer is desired, which may be unattainable by some with limited budgets. Research by

Barker-Ruchti *et al.* (2021), discussing that financial limitations are likely to lead to reallocation of funds from other areas and a potential disadvantage. They go on to discuss that one such disadvantage might be financing technologies in a men's side will further disadvantage areas with less funding already such as women's sides and participation-level sport. Other research tends to agree with Baerg (2017) arguing that technological costs create a digital divide and amplify inequalities. Given the increased availability, knowledge and often aggressive marketing strategies of technology companies, pressure builds to invest which may lead to consequential decision making and financial troubles if not managed carefully. Further, given the abundant number of technologies now available for procurement, it can become somewhat overwhelming to know which to invest in and also requires those who are making decisions to have relevant knowledge to understand differences in different analysis technologies and the cost versus benefit they each provide (Luczak *et al.*, 2020). It is therefore clear that in a technologically rich and complicated marketplace, solutions are required to provide support for decision making and wise investment into the right technologies for the environment.

Parallel Solutions and Workflow Examples

Whilst it is true that our discipline area is rich with technological options, analysts need not always elect for the expensive option, especially if working on budgetary constraints. As this chapter continues, we're going to consider applied examples where performance analysis workflows are typically used to provide support for the coaching process, information for end-users and ultimately help enhance performance. As we do so, we'll consider the different options available technologically to help support these needs, assessing the viability, pros and cons of differently priced (or free) technologies. It is anticipated that this content will be considered critically in tandem with that from Chapter 2 which outlined and detailed many of the functionalities of the technologies now available. Meanwhile provide examples of comparative technologies for the same purposes, some pros and cons and importantly, the price points of each. These technological solutions are by no means exhaustive, nor a direct endorsement of any and prices are indicative only in GBP. It is hoped that this content will respond to the research of Luczak *et al.* (2020) and others, by providing informed work to allow stakeholders to make more informed decisions and wise investments.

Scenario 1: Pre-match

Commonplace in most analysis departments, the role of pre-match analysis is to help players become more informed about their own and oppositions game to be more prepared for upcoming matches (Fernandez-Echeverria *et al.*, 2019). It is anticipated by Groom and Cushion (2004) that this leads to an opportunity to develop an effective style of play for that upcoming game. In this phase the use of video and data from either internal or external sources is required in order to assess visually and quantitatively the areas of strength and weakness. Some settings report limited access to this with 33% without video and 54% without data in Andersen *et al.*'s (2022) football-based study, and so parallel solutions for all price points to enable this are required.

Data gathering and insights where money is not an object sees this largely outsourced to specialist companies and data providers under strict contractual clauses. The raw data is collected by the company's in-house teams before being provided back to the user by raw files, statistics, rankings and infographics for which an annual subscription is typically negotiated. An ongoing issue with such data sources however is reliability, with several conflicting numbers found when directly correlating multiple data providers on the same events in the same matches. Data sources are most prevalent in football, though many also exist in other sports including tennis, rugby union and netball. Where full data purchase is not feasible, analysts will have to look elsewhere to garner data-driven insights into performances. One option would be to procure access to only the teams and leagues required for a single user, rather than an all-encompassing worldwide access. Failing that, then some companies offer significant data sets for certain leagues and competitions as open source, meaning anyone can access and utilise free of charge. In match meanwhile many broadcasters will produce certain data too which can be harvested, though again some issues with definition and reliability may remain. Working on the premise of an exceptionally small or non-existent budget makes data analysis processes harder to undertake, but far from impossible. It is likely that even open source data will not be useful here since the level at which there is no budget at all will be much lower, and not covered by the commercial companies. Therefore, all data will need to be generated in house and most likely fall to a placement or internship student to code. This manual generation will be time consuming however and rely on access to video being present to enable coding to take place.

Once collated the data that is ready for processing will need to be entered into a software to produce insights, elite workflows will see this entered in raw formats to powerful data processing software such as Tableau or PowerBI bought for multiple users, which allow personalised visualisations, reporting and analysis of the core data. For a lower cost solution, individual licences procured for single users may be possible or through a placement student or internship students university subscription. Standard to most computers, Excel or Numbers may be used as a low to no-cost alternative, albeit with lesser functions, whilst some may also make the most of free trials on multiple machines. It should also be noted that the specialist nature of the more powerful software will likely require a specialist to be recruited, or existing member upskilled, incurring wages and costs.

Video of opposition is typically accessed via commercial sites such as WyScout for football (Figure 10.1), subscriptions to paywall protected content, or via

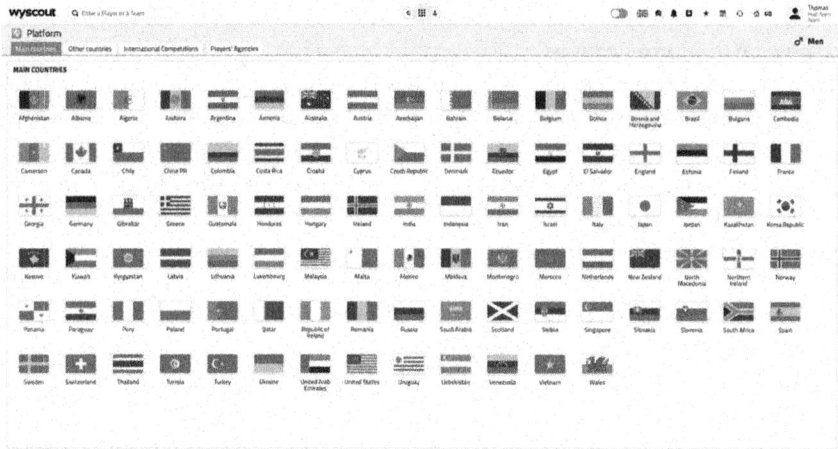

FIGURE 10.1 WyScout.

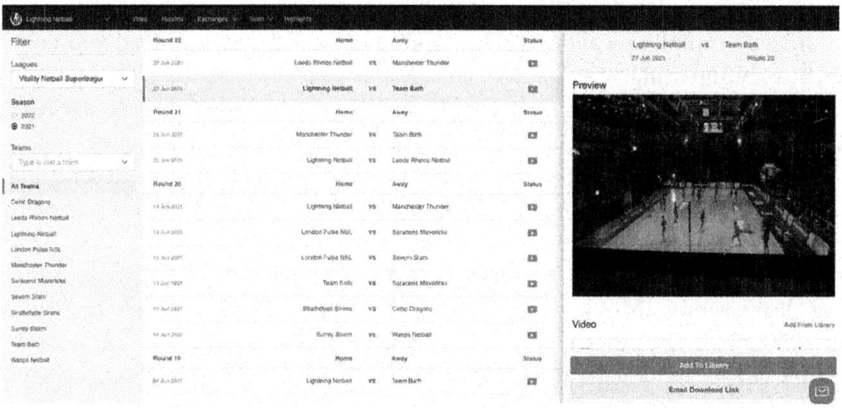

FIGURE 10.2 Hudl league exchange.

league-wide reciprocal sharing agreements in sports such as rugby union (via Elite-Hub) and netball (via Hudl League Exchange, see Figure 10.2) which allow opposition to access full match videos of any other team in the league. As with data access, organisations may opt to purchase single league or club accounts of commercial providers to gain crucial opposition footage at a lower cost. Failing that, there may be a league exchange agreement in place even if not on a platform such as Hudl but instead on shared folders. If not, then reciprocal direct swaps for footage with other teams' analysts may be negotiated instead to provide some footage. Beyond this, footage can be gathered in more creative ways, screen capturing through QuickTime any footage that is streamed online including on social media, opting for broadcast highlights or attending opposition games and filming where permitted, though recognising the limits this brings and potential permissions and implications.

To process and analyse the video once gathered, an analysis software will be needed to enter the raw files and then pull out important clips and data (e.g. SportsCode, Catapult Pro Video – Focus, Angles and NacSport), alongside telestration tools (e.g. Studio and Coach Paint) to graphically illustrate important areas of attention in elite workflows. These will then be outputted into high-end presentations through the analysis software themselves or into Key-Note, Prezi or PowerPoint for delivery in person or online hosting on Hudl. com (or similar) and sending directly such as via WhatsApp. For lower budgets, there are now several viable alternatives to the main software providers, offering similar functionality at a fraction of the price, as per Table 10.1. Where this is still not possible, some offer free versions (e.g. Longomatch and Kinovea), or reverting back to raw video files in QuickTime player and noting times down manually to drag to when needed is a longer and less flashy, but workable solution. That footage could still be clipped and then hosted on a free private YouTube channel, a DropBox or OneDrive account to ensure that work can be shared with players and staff alike and offer remote communicative options such as commenting.

For telestration, if not already included in the analysis software package, additional software fees can be avoided entirely by purchasing one of the excellent multipurpose Logitech Spotlight remotes, which ably assist in highlighting areas of interest, alongside play/pause and zoom capabilities, though these would only work for live delivery and not online hosting of video. After this, then using the basic freeze frame, zoom, crop and drawing tools ensuring clear opacity, iMovie software which is native to all new Apple machines delivers a basic but useful solution for telestration (see Figure 10.3), as to do simple shape drawings over video in PowerPoint. Or users might opt to use the remote functionality of Apple's presentation software KeyNote, which allows for simple drawings to be added on top of presentations, including over video.

Regarding personnel, high-end settings will see analysts employed full time, typically with a job role solely associated with this pre-match phase and perhaps with the assistance of a paid placement student. With lower budgets, it is likely that a full-time analyst will still be employed; however, their remit will be much wider, covering all phases of analysis rather than specialising and assisted by a number of paid placement or internship students. With no budget for full- or part-time staff, unless opting for a very low paid or worse still unpaid student intern, there may be a need to shift responsibility for analysis towards an assistant coach or the head coach themselves to drive this provision which may serve as a valuable learning and upskilling tool as part of a coach's ongoing development. Organisations might also make use of injured players, parents, supporters or media teams to help with some provision and editing too.

TABLE 10.1 Software options

Item	Possible providers	Pros	Cons	Indicative cost
Data provider	WyScout Opta InStat StatsBomb Champion Data	– Speed and convenience. – Automated reports and analysis. – Opposition access and scouting.	– Validity/reliability. – Consistency of definitions. – Contractual clauses/usage limits.	Full access: £6,000–£10,000. Per year, per licence.
	Broadcaster	– Data harvesting from existing source. – Access to opposition data.	– Limited data points. – Validity/reliability. – Inconsistency/limited access.	£0.
	Open Source	– Substantial data points. – Speed and convenience of access.	– Requires programming knowledge. – Limited leagues/players available.	£0.
	Manual Coding	– Bespoke collection of exact indicators for each team/athlete. – In-house definitions and reliability.	– Time consuming. – Reliant on suitable video access.	£0.
Data processor	Tableau PowerBi IBM Cognos Oracle Cloud Sisense	– Automated and personalised report building. – Data handling efficiency with large volumes. – Cloud hosted security.	– Data hosting limits. – Restrictive data imports. – Scaling cost to all staff.	£200–£800. Per year, per licence.
	Excel Numbers	– Pre-install on most new machines. – Simple report generation. – Familiarity and ease of use.	– Limited data import capacity. – Limited range of analytical tools and visualisations.	£0.
Video provider	WyScout Opta	– Professional video of multiple teams. – Speed of access.	– Limited sports only.	Full access: £2,000+ Per year, per licence.
	Streaming Services	– Access to international leagues.	– Availability and access not guaranteed. – Licencing and legal considerations.	Varied.

(Continued)

Item	Possible providers	Pros	Cons	Indicative cost
	League Sharing Agreements	– League-wide access to opposition. – Reciprocal agreements.	– Lower quality footage. – Relying on opposition to conform to upload agreements.	
	Direct Swaps	– Instant access when agreed. – Develop relations for future swaps.	– Not widely accessible. – Relies on mutual agreements.	£0.
	Social Media Broadcaster	– Recording from existing sources. – Access to opposition footage.	– Limited quality. – Limited length and duration. – Inconsistency/limited access.	
Analysis software	SportsCode Elite SBG Focus Angles NacSport	– Ingests video and some data types for analysis. – Time stamped events.	– Some integration issues. – Requires expert user to operate.	£400–£2,000. Per year, per licence.
	Longomatch Kinovea	– Produces clipped footage for analysis sessions.	– Limited functionality. – Limited file type acceptance.	Free–£500. Per year, per licence.
	QuickTime iMovie/Movie Maker	– Simple video clipping.	– Non-bespoke software. – Time consuming and manual process.	Included on most new machines.
Telestration software	Studio Coach Paint Metrica Play KlipDraw	– Dynamic illustrations on video footage. – Enhances learning and attention. – Aids retention and engagement.	– Time consuming to create. – Some integration issues.	£65–£5,000. Per year, per licence.
	Logitech Spotlight Remote	– Multipurpose portable remote. – Highlights, zooms and pauses.	– Manually operated as presenting live. – Live use only, no pre-programmed.	£140.
	iMovie PowerPoint/ KeyNote	– Simple highlighting and drawings.	– Non-bespoke software. – Basic features only.	Included on most new machines.

	Item	Advantages	Disadvantages	Cost
Present	Analysis Software	– Single software fully integrated.	– Less control of look and feel.	As above.
	KeyNote			Included on most new machines.
	PowerPoint	– Dynamic presentations. – Interactive elements. – Cloud hosted possibilities.	– Limited integration. – Time consuming creation and transfer.	£60–£720. Per year, per licence.
	Prezi			
Radio contact	Irisun Pro	– Professional quality. – Portable, multi-use for training and match days.	– Prone to interference. – May require permissions to use at some venues.	£600. Pack of 6.
	CPS Telecom Compact	– Space saving. – Small to fit in pockets.	– Less powerful. – Prone to interference/cross talk.	£70 each.
	Zello	– App-based, no hardware required. – Simple to use and reliable. – Playback feature to re-listen to messages.	– Relies on internet connection. – Needs personal or company phone.	Free
Human resource	Dedicated Pre-Match Analyst General Analyst	– Qualified analyst dedicated to the role(s). – Expertise to aid preparation. – Interaction and contribution to the IDT.	– None.	£25,000+. Per year.
	Placement Student Internship Student	– Willingness and eager. – Contemporary knowledge. – Educational alignment.	– Less/no experience. – Require more time to complete tasks. – Academic time commitments.	£0–£10,000. Per year. £0–minimum wage per hour.
	Assistant Coach/ Head Coach	– Deep knowledge of game/tactics. – Alignment with coaching delivery.	– Time consuming. – Takes away from main role.	Varied.
Total			circa.	£1,000–£100,000

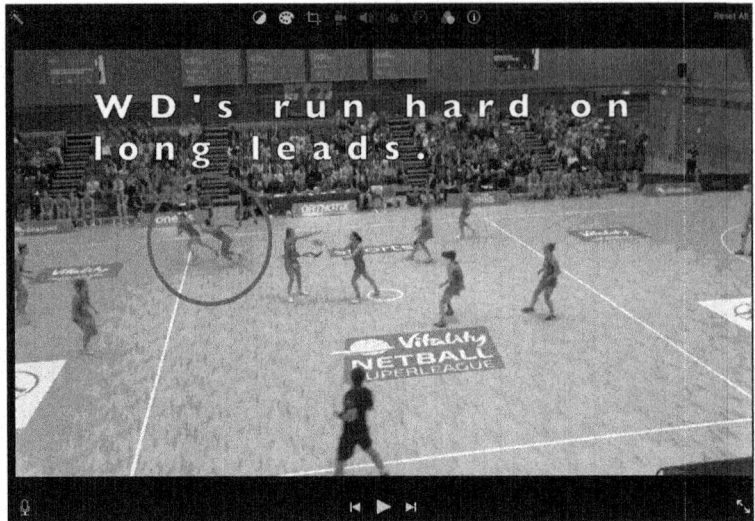

FIGURE 10.3   Manual telestration.

Scenario 2: Training Analysis

The capture, coding and analysis of training events is now well embedded in most sports. The findings elicited from pre-match analysis work should have a direct influence on the training practice, correlating what was found in pre-match to design and rehearse appropriate tactical responses. Utilising the pre-match findings to directly inform coaching practice in the days leading up to the match is an important step and ensures that the training week is designed appropriately. The maintenance and analysis of the players responses and actions to these is critical in developing tactics and technical competencies before the match itself. Feeding back those training events via filming, coding and analysis either in- or post-session allows for holistic conversations and for the fine tuning of performance.

In training sessions, elite environments with ample funds will typically see training captured live by an analyst who simultaneously codes critical incidents, before facilitating live in- and post-session replay opportunities. In order to provide this a first consideration is the filming vantage point with natural height from nearby structures or balconies an advantage where possible, with investment into permanent IP cameras to stream footage back to a dedicated point the ideal, though expensive solution. In more temperate budgets, portable filming masts such as the EndZone systems allow for heightened filming angles and will work on multiple different training areas. Aside from this, those with exceptionally low or no budgets will have to make do with floor level filming, or attempt to fix camera equipment to tables or other structures in the vicinity, in the safest way they can. Elite cameras will be 4K resolution or better akin to broadcast equipment, though standard HD cameras can do just as good job on lower budgets, with some exceptionally reasonable alternatives available as listed in Table 10.2.

TABLE 10.2 Hardware options

Item		Possible providers	Pros	Cons	Indicative cost
Camera		Fixed IP Cameras	– Professional quality video capture. – Consistent positioning and location. – Wired link back to set location. – Some with AI-enabled tracking.	– Non-portable limits other uses. – Some systems require software install.	£5,000+ Per camera.
		Canon XA45 4K	– Portable, high quality – Multi-use in different phases. – Consistent output and compatibility with capture devices.	– Manually operated.	£1,400. Per camera.
		Canon Legria HFG40 UHD	– Portable, high quality – Multi-use in different phases. – Consistent output and compatibility with capture devices.	– Manually operated. – Slightly lower quality.	£900. Per camera.
		Canon Legria HF R86 HD	– Portable, compact camera. – Multi-use in different phases.	– Manually operated. – Lower quality, less powerful.	£300. Per camera.
		EndZone Telescoping Tower	– Gains filming height where natural vantage point not present. – Portable to use on multiple areas.	– Bulky and awkward to transport. – Time consuming to set up.	£2,500+ Per tower.
Conversion device		BlackMagic	– Ingest multiple video input types.	– Requires software install on capture device. – Not widely supported by software companies.	£110.
		AJA U-Tap	– Plug and play. – No software required.	– None.	£400.

(Continued)

Item	Possible providers	Pros	Cons	Indicative cost
Projection	Bespoke Golf Carts	– Bespoke solution for outdoor environments. – Portable use on multiple spaces.	– Storage issues. – Power limited.	£8,000+.
	Ultra Short Throw	– Powerful device for compact areas. – Very large picture output. – Portable multi-use.	– Can be noisy/excude heat.	£1,200+.
	4K/UHD	– High quality output device. – Portable multi-use.	– Requires space to project across room.	£500–£1,000.
	Standard	– Suitable output device. – Portable multi-use.	– Lower quality. – Requires space to project across room.	£200–£500.
	TV Screen	– Fixed permanent solution.	– Non-portable, limiting usefulness.	£300–£800.
	Ruckus	– Powerful long range indoor/outdoor solution. – Able to carry volumes of data wirelessly.	– Time consuming set up. – Reliability issues in dense environments. – May require multiple devices to connect.	£400–£1,200. Per device, depending on range.

	NetGear Nighthawk Router	– Shorter range indoor solution. – Quick and easy set up.	– Shorter range. – Reliability issues in dense environments.	£250–£500.
	Hard Wired/Switches	– Hard wired physical connection. – Reliable. – Can carry large volumes of data.	– Physical wiring set up required. – Non-portable solution.	Varied.
Computer	MacBook Pro	– Portable and multi-use.	– Most expensive. – Small screen size.	£2,399–£3,299. Per machine.
	Mac Mini	– Space saving.	– Less powerful. - Requires external monitor.	£700–£1,099. Per machine.
	iMac	– Powerful permanent solution.	– Non-portable limits other uses.	£1,249–£1,649. Per machine.
	iPad Pro	– Powerful device for receiving video. – Portable, multipurpose.	– Limited connectivity.	£749–£999
	Windows PC	– Multipurpose.	– Most analysis software are Mac only. – Limited compatibility. – Less powerful.	£400–£2,000. Per machine.
Total			circa.	£1,000–£100,000

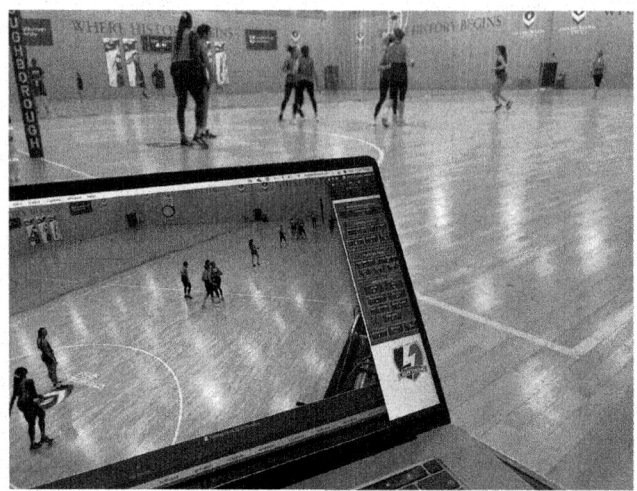

FIGURE 10.4 Live replay in training.

Where possible, live output video feeds from the cameras will be inputted into Mac based hardware (as per pre-match technologies above) via BlackMagic Design or AJA U-Tap convertor boxes, before being ingested into an analysis software for coding. Assuming this is possible, the projection of training is then sent out to another fully licensed machine via networking devices attached to fixed or portable big screens and projectors, with outdoor environments some-times using specially created golf carts with screens on to enable review. This near instant replay of training allows and stimulates critical conversation about training practices, allows opportunities to identify fixes and promotes athlete self-engagement with analysis. If a projector cannot be procured, then viewing footage on a standard television screen mounted to a wall connected with HDMI will suit, or on a laptop screen providing ample opportunity for engagement with training analysis in the moment (see Figure 10.4).

For those who cannot invest in the full live replay technologies to enable this, using a single machine to capture onto and then review will save considerable money on additional Mac devices, software licences and networking equipment. In such instances, ingesting the feed is still required via convertor devices and into a single licenced analysis machine. This machine can then be directly taken to athletes to view back instances straight away rather than investing into a pro-jection device or if the filming vantage point is close enough, asking athletes to move to there. Beyond this, if live capture equipment is too pricey, then it will be critical that training is filmed with one of the identified cameras and footage then downloaded post-training to enable upload to a video hosting platform (e.g. Hudl.com, DropBox and OneDrive) for conversation, commenting and re-view. Other alternatives include filming on tablet devices such as iPads, which then allow for instant replay back and potential connection to projectors, though quality will be lower and this is a manually intensive process, alternatively two iPads would enable filming from one, with a Zoom, FaceTime or similar call set up to the other acting as a review tool. Those with ample money may employ a specialist training analyst responsible for all areas of delivery, potentially with the support of student analysts. A generic all-encompassing analyst (as per pre-match) may be used elsewhere, or a reliance on students where money is an object. With no support, asking injured players or other support staff to film would be beneficial, failing that then leaving cameras static over play for post-session upload would be a solution, to save pulling an assistant coach out of their coaching role to enable this.

Scenario 3: Match Analysis

The most commonly used of all workflows, match analysis is widely recognised as vital for success. The collection of video and data of incidents and events throughout the match allows for decisions to be made and in some environments this happens simultaneously. The efficacious use of this analysis workflow provides the opportunity for monitoring and evaluation with a view to improving performance (Hughes & Bartlett, 2002). Other research suggests that in certain sports, football in this case, 79% of analysts are involved in some form of live data capture and analysis. Given this significant number, it is perhaps not surprising that this is deemed such a vital cog in the coaching process.

As per Table 10.2, much of the equipment required for a matchday is replicated from that of training, with elite environments using multiple machines networked together to provide review stations for analysts or coaches in the moment, and additional devices set in changing rooms for review during half-time breaks, perhaps presented on an interactive screen or via an ultra-short throw projector. IP camera feeds and broadcast footage are likely to be ingested into multiple powerful hardware devices simultaneously to deliver excellent video angles for quick review. Even if a third-party data provider is used for data access from matches, many will still complete their own coding in match to attain to coaching needs and for accuracy of definition (Wright *et al.,* 2013). And so, the use of collaborative coding by multiple analysts on match days is common, with often two or more analysts coding onto their own respective machines, in addition to one filming a wide angle for review, which sync back to another machine for full review by perhaps an assistant coach. This maintains quality of live capture, code and review but does require an ability to multitask in real time in high pressure scenarios. Communication of that back in the moment to the coaches delivering instructions might be via high-end radios (though consideration must be paid to licencing if building a large network of devices) or integrated stadium phones, but more likely via Wi-Fi-enabled apps such as Zello, a free product.

Without an ability to invest in multiple machines and licences, users will have to consider alternative means by which to undertake their analysis. Having a lower quality camera, single MacBook and licence will considerably lower the cost, whilst still providing a strong workflow for review. This single machine could still provide a video and statistical output window to the bench via a simple screen share on Zoom or similar over reliable stadium Wi-Fi or a personal hotspot, allowing insights in match for the staff delivering instructions. Further savings could be made with the type of licence, with a possibility being to film the match to a memory card and then code the game afterwards meaning a cheaper review licence could be purchased rather than an elite live capture one, if using Hudl products, though this of course precludes and live data or video being presented in game. If that remains a priority, then a very simple yet effective manual workflow would be to notate events by hand and the time in game they happened, then quickly transfer the first half footage onto a laptop for changing room review, before manually moving the timestamp to find passages of play of interest to present back. Alternative projection ideas include using only the laptop screen itself with no additional cost, a more basic entry-level projector or TV screens which may already be mounted in venue.

Scenario 4: Post-match Analysis

After performances have been completed, post-match analysis allows an opportunity to reflect upon the events, in line with pre-match expectations and plans. The structure and timings of sessions is critical, allowing suitable time for emotions to subside whilst simultaneously providing opportunity for objective analysis content and athlete input. Post-match debriefing involves two stages for analysts; preparation and presentation. In many scenarios, analysts will undertake the former, but less often the latter with coaches taking the lead instead. The use of video, data and additional interactive tools such as telestration are commonplace here, to aid retention and takeaway messages before the next iteration begins (Jones *et al.*, 2020).

Post-match technologies are largely made up of those used elsewhere so far, with immediate post-match analysis beginning for the analyst with the upload of video and coding to a storage site immediately post-match. For most, this will be elite sites such as Hudl.com or Catapult Pro Video – Hub, though private YouTube channels, OneDrive and DropBox offer alternative solutions too. The analysts might also send output window reports of initial key numbers that help attain to pre-match plans and tactical desires, and assess the level to which the team or individuals successfully completed their roles. This may be sent via the online storage site, or more commonly through instant messaging services such as WhatsApp. For those not able to code live, this process will usually be completed soon after, and then the same sharing methods utilised. Additional coding might be completed by some, which will be done to enable a deeper review and individualised reporting, though this laborious process will only be required if data access has not been purchased previously, and so will largely happen with those on smaller budgets. They might seek to utilise student placements for this key developmental activity, or elect to focus only on team and unit-based numbers instead.

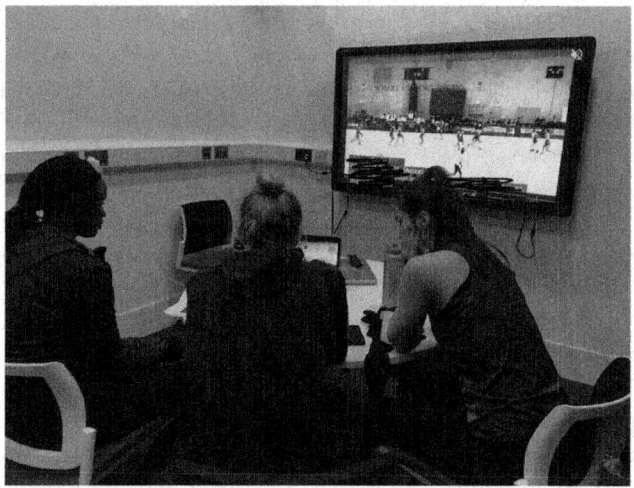

FIGURE 10.5 Athlete–led unit debrief.

With a suggested delay of 24–48 hours to allow emotions to subside for a more objective and unbiased look back at the game, debriefing delivery will then take place. Approaches here vary, with some coaches taking the lead and using materials prepared by the analysts or in conjunction with them to deliver directly. More recent trends have seen analysts themselves deliver to players, and though the most recent research into this (e.g. Wright *et al.*, 2013) suggests only 13% of analysts deliver to players, anecdotally this number is now increasing as trust and the role of the analyst increase. More common also is the use of athlete led debriefs, tasking them with the responsibility to discuss and find solutions to periods of the match themselves before sharing back to the group (see Figure 10.5). Whichever option is elected for, it is likely that telestration will be used in some form, and so the solutions presented in pre-match and Table 10.1, will again be required. As too will a form of large screen to display, with many bespoke environments having purpose-built rooms or projectors for this. Others will opt for portable devices such as ultra-short throw projectors or more traditional ones which are reasonable and multi-use for the various phases of an analysis cycle. Failing this then lower budgets might seek to use club room or function rooms with pre-installed televisions, or seek to purchase a very low-cost television to use for this purpose.

Technological Consequences and Decision Making

The role, place and importance of performance analysis are now firmly embedded, with significant research evidence to highlight the positive role it plays in helping enhance the outcomes of performances at developmental and performance level. Many allow the analyst(s) to *actually analyse* rather than spending considerable time in manually capturing and coding performances before that process can begin. They speed up workflows considerably and allow for earlier planning and more advanced discussions ahead of upcoming matches, or for more informed decisions in match and more efficient debriefs. There is of course no guarantee of successes if investment is made given the vast number of contextual factors that influence the outcome of sporting performances, and so for those who are not in a strong fiscal position, a difficult conundrum arises as they seek to balance the relative necessity of an analysis provision, with finding and investing some form of finances towards it.

Analysts and coaches alike may promote the usefulness in practice, but those holding budgetary responsibility will be the ultimate decision makers. This might result in full, some or no provision being procured for use. So, in putting forwards budget requests, analysts should very carefully consider the total monies they are working within and the relative functionality that various pieces of equipment will provide them. Adopting information from this chapter, decision makers need to decide upon which blend of technologies they require and can afford from the three options showcased in each workflow phase here weighing up a cost-benefit analysis for performance impact. Some may *double up* from the different analysis phases and have multiple uses, e.g. the pre-match analysts MacBook might also be used on a match day, although in the high-end workflows multiple machines with multiple licences are going to be required. These and all other investment decisions should be based on need to haves, not nice to haves and must be carefully considered with a pedagogical approach in mind. So, whilst a fully automated AI-enabled IP camera set for each pitch and the stadium might be nice to have, manually operated PTZ cameras that cover multiple pitches may be a more cost-effective solution. After all, do you really *need* it to automatically track play for you and will you be 100% happy with the angles and tracking accuracy produced? Or perhaps a manually operated joystick PTZ camera will provide extremely valuable experience for a paid placement student to learn their craft, whilst also delivering quality footage for entry into another live capture licences, which might otherwise not have been possible if the AI-enabled option were taken.

Performance analysis can be an expensive discipline to invest in, but it need not be restrictive and a barrier if sensible and well-informed decisions are made. A key part of the analyst's job in lower functionality environments will be to help communicate back to the end users that turnaround times may be longer, due to more manual coding and analysis being employed. There will therefore have to be an acceptance that functionality will not be as high, or as quick, but still operational and useable in the coaching process. Carefully thinking this through and providing clear just reasoning with clear prioritisation areas in mind may help allow for analysis to benefit from wider investments. And so now if a lower-league team want to analyse their own matches with the use of technology, they will have options to invest in reasonably priced cameras, a coding software that is functional on multiple machines and presentation software that allows for delivery of important messages with basic telestration.

Concluding Remarks

With an analyst's kit bags more often than not resembling a high-street technology store, it is not hard to see how costs can significantly spiral. With the place of performance analysis so firmly embedded in the armoury of most environments, there is a need to invest wisely in equipment to allow for provision. The breadth and depth of products on offer now has done little to drive down prices, with the most functional technologies remaining stubbornly expensive. With newer, faster and more automated technologies continuing to be developed, promising more time for *actual analysis*, the upward curve in technology (and price) looks set to continue. For some this will mean little or no investment can be made, as the prices preclude budgetary confines and economic shortfalls, no matter the desire. In time, more products are likely to come to the mass market with lower prices, but until then, alternatives must be sought.

The good news is that these do exist, as highlighted in this chapter, and they do allow for processes to be implemented and provision to be provided. Taking time to carefully consider cost effective solutions which meet the needs of end users in a timely manner is a critical stage for any analyst, perhaps none more so than those with much smaller budgets. In doing so, analysts must of course bear in mind that the functionality might not be as high as the market leaders, but be safe in the knowledge that they have made sensible informed decisions to provide the best they can, in the environment under which they operate. For all practitioners, no matter the budget, the importance of process over product and the pedagogical impacts of learning technologies should be at the centre of any decision making. If so, the future of applied performance analysis looks set to continue as an exciting, dynamic and informative discipline.

References

Andersen, L.W., Francis, J.W., & Bateman, M. (2022). Danish association football coaches' perception of performance analysis. *International Journal of Performance Analysis in Sport, 22*(1), 149–173.

Baerg, A. (2017). Big data, sport and the digital divide: Theorizing how athletes might respond to big data monitoring. *Journal of Sport and Social Issues, 41*(1), 3–20.

Barker-Ruchti, N., Svensson, R., Svensson, D., & Fransson, D. (2021). Don't buy a pig in a poke: Considering challenges of and problems with performance analysis technologies in Swedish men's elite football. *Performance Enhancement & Health, 9*(1), 100191.

Fernandez-Echeverria, C., Mesquita, I., Conejero, M., & Moreno, M.P. (2019). Perceptions of elite volleyball players on the importance of match analysis during the training process. *International Journal of Performance Analysis in Sport, 19*(1), 49–64.

Groom, R., & Cushion, C. (2004). Coaches perceptions of the use of video analysis: A case study. *Insight, 7*(3), 56–58.

Hughes, M.D., & Bartlett, R.M. (2002). The use of performance indicators in performance analysis. *Journal of Sports Sciences, 20*, 739–754.

Jones, D., Rands, S., & Butterworth, A.D. (2020). The use and perceived value of telestration tools in elite football. *International Journal of Performance Analysis in Sport, 20*(3), 373–388.

Luczak, T., Burch, R., Lewis, E., Chandler, H., & Ball, J. (2020). State-of-the-art review of athletic wearable technology: What 113 strength and conditioning coaches and athletic trainers from USA said about technology in sports. *International Journal of Sports Science & Coaching, 15*(1), 26–40.

Wright, C., Atkins, S., Jones, B., & Todd, J. (2013). The role of performance analysts within the coaching process: Performance Analysts Survey 'The role of performance analysts in elite football club settings.' *International Journal of Performance Analysis in Sport, 13*(1), 240–261.

INDEX